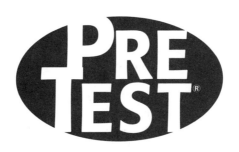

Pharmacology

PreTest® Self-Assessment and Review

Notice

Medicine is an ever-changing science. As new research and clinical experience broaden our knowledge, changes in treatment and drug therapy are required. The authors and the publisher of this work have checked with sources believed to be reliable in their efforts to provide information that is complete and generally in accord with the standards accepted at the time of publication. However, in view of the possibility of human error or changes in medical sciences, neither the authors nor the publisher nor any other party who has been involved in the preparation or publication of this work warrants that the information contained herein is in every respect accurate or complete, and they disclaim all responsibility for any errors or omissions or for the results obtained from use of the information contained in this work. Readers are encouraged to confirm the information contained herein with other sources. For example and in particular, readers are advised to check the product information sheet included in the package of each drug they plan to administer to be certain that the information contained in this work is accurate and that changes have not been made in the recommended dose or in the contraindications for administration. This recommendation is of particular importance in connection with new or infrequently used drugs.

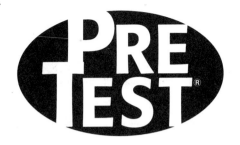

Pharmacology
PreTest® Self-Assessment and Review
Tenth Edition

Arnold Stern, M.D., Ph.D.
Professor of Pharmacology
Department of Pharmacology
New York University School of Medicine
New York, New York

Student Reviewers
Christopher A. Heck
University of South Alabama College of Medicine
Mobile, Alabama
Class of 2001

Junda C. Woo
State University of New York at Buffalo School of Medicine and Biomedical Sciences
Buffalo, New York
Class of 2002

McGraw-Hill
Medical Publishing Division
New York   Chicago   San Francisco   Lisbon   London   Madrid   Mexico City
Milan   New Delhi   San Juan   Seoul   Singapore   Sydney   Toronto

McGraw-Hill

A Division of The McGraw-Hill Companies

Pharmacology: PreTest® Self-Assessment and Review, Tenth Edition

Copyright © 2002 by The **McGraw-Hill Companies**, Inc. All rights reserved. Printed in the United States of America. Except as permitted under the United States Copyright Act of 1976, no part of this publication may be reproduced or distributed in any form or by any means, or stored in a data base or retrieval system, without the prior written permission of the publisher.

Previous editions copyright © 1999, 1996, 1993, 1991, 1988, 1986, 1983, 1980, and 1976 by The McGraw-Hill Companies, Inc.

2 3 4 5 6 7 8 9 0 DOC/DOC 0 9 8 7 6 5 4 3 2

ISBN 0-07-136704-7

This book was set in Berkeley by North Market Street Graphics.
The editor was Catherine A. Johnson.
The production supervisor was Phil Galea.
Project management was provided by North Market Street Graphics.
The cover designer was Li Chen Chang/Pinpoint.
R.R. Donnelley & Sons was printer and binder.

This book is printed on acid-free paper.

Library of Congress Cataloging-in-Publication Data

Pharmacology: PreTest self-assessment and review.—10th ed. / [edited by] Arnold Stern; student reviewers, Christopher A. Heck, Junda C. Woo.
    p. ; cm.
    Includes bibliographical references and index.
    ISBN 0-07-136704-7 (alk. paper)
        1. Pharmacology—Examinations, questions, etc.   2. Physicians—Licenses—United States—Examinations—Study guides.   I. Stern, Arnold.
        [DNLM: 1. Pharmacology—Examination Questions. QV 18.2 P536 2001]
    RM301.13.P475 2001
    615'.1'076—dc21   2001034253

Contents

High-Yield Facts

General Principles

Anti-Infectives

Cancer Chemotherapy and Immunology

Cardiovascular and Pulmonary Systems

Central Nervous System

Autonomic Nervous System

Local Control Substances

Renal System

Gastrointestinal System and Nutrition

Endocrine System

Toxicology

Preface

In this tenth edition of *Pharmacology: PreTest® Self-Assessment and Review,* significant changes and improvements have been made. Questions that use clinical vignettes have been added; the responses require interpretation and data synthesis. The number of items per group of matching questions has been reduced in accordance with the new format used on United States Medical Licensing Examination (USMLE) Step 1. A High-Yield Facts section containing two sample Drug Classification Tables has been added; these tables serve as simple examples for collating and comparing information about various drug classes. References have been updated, and this section is preceded by a List of Abbreviations and Acronyms used throughout the book.

The author remains indebted to his students and colleagues at New York University Medical Center for their continuing support and encouragement.

Introduction

Each *PreTest® Self-Assessment and Review* allows medical students to comprehensively and conveniently assess and review their knowledge of a particular basic science—in this instance, pharmacology. The 490 questions parallel the format and degree of difficulty of the questions found in the United States Medical Licensing Examination (USMLE) Step 1. Practicing physicians who want to hone their skills before USMLE Step 3 or recertification may find this to be a good beginning in their review process.

Each question is accompanied by an answer, a paragraph explanation, and a specific page reference to an appropriate textbook. A bibliography listing sources can be found following the last chapter.

Before each chapter, a list of key terms or classifications of drugs or both is included to aid review. In addition, suggestions for effective study and review have been added afterward.

The most effective method of using this book is to complete one chapter at a time. Prepare yourself for each chapter by reviewing from your notes and favorite text the drugs classes listed at the beginning of each section and the drugs listed in the "High-Yield Facts" section. You should concentrate especially on the prototype drugs. Then proceed to indicate your answer by each question, allowing yourself not more than one minute for each question. In this way you will be approximating the time limits imposed by the examination.

After you finish going through the questions in the section, spend as much time as you need verifying your answers and carefully reading the explanations provided. Pay special attention to the explanations for the questions you answered incorrectly—but read *every* explanation. The editors of this material have designed the explanations to reinforce and supplement the information tested by the questions. If you feel you need further information about the material covered, consult and study the references indicated.

High-Yield Facts

SAMPLE DRUG CLASSIFICATION TABLES

TIPS FOR LEARNING PHARMACOLOGY

Pharmacology is best learned by comparing drugs within a particular class or by their specific use.

A chart highlighting the similarities and differences among the various agents can be a helpful tool. The charts included in this section are simple examples. More elaborate charts can be constructed that would include how the drug is administered, its pharmacological effects, its adverse effects, its mechanism of toxicity (if known), and significant drug-drug interactions. For infectious disease agents, the spectrum of antimicrobial activity and the basis of antibiotic resistance can be added.

Explanations for the abbreviations used in these charts are found in the List of Abbreviations and Acronyms, which appears before the Bibliography.

Drugs for Treating Bacterial Infectious Diseases

Drug Class	Prototype	Action	Spectrum
Penicillins		Inhibit bacterial cell-wall synthesis by binding to penicillin-binding proteins, inhibiting crosslinking enzymes, and activating autolytic enzymes that disrupt bacterial cell walls.	Streptococci, meningococci, pneumococci, gram-positive bacilli, gonococci, spirochetes.
Narrow spectrum			
Penicillinase-susceptible	Penicillin G		
Penicillinase-resistant	Methicillin		Staphylococci.
Wide spectrum	Ampicillin		Similar to penicillin G; also includes *E. coli, P mirabilis,* and *H. influenzae.*
Penicillinase-susceptible	Carbenicillin		Gram-negative rods and especially useful for *Pseudomonas* spp.
Cephalosporins			
First-generation	Cephalothin		Gram-positive cocci, *E. coli,* and *K. pneumoniae.*
Second-generation	Cefamandole		Greater activity against gram-negative organisms than first-generation cephalosporins.
Third-generation	Cefoperazone		Broader activity against resistant gram-negative organisms; some derivatives penetrate the blood-brain barrier.
Carbapenem	Imipenem		Wide action against gram-positive cocci, gram-negative rods, and some anaerobes.
Monobactam	Aztreonam		Resistant to β-lactamases produced by gram-negative rods.

Drug	Mechanism	Spectrum
Macrolides		
Erythromycin	Inhibits protein synthesis by binding to part of the 50S ribosomal subunit	Gram-positive cocci, mycoplasma, corynebacteria, *Legionella*, *Ureaplasma*, *Bordetella*.
Vancomycin	Inhibits synthesis of cell-wall mucopeptides (peptidoglycans).	Gram-positive bacteria, especially for resistant mutants.
Chloramphenicol	Inhibits peptide bond formation by binding to the 50S ribosomal subunit, inhibiting peptidyl transferase.	*Salmonella* and *Haemophilus* infections and meningococcal and pneumococcal meningitis.
Aminoglycosides		
Systemic		
Gentamicin	Inhibits protein synthesis by binding to the 30S subunit of ribosomes, which blocks formation of the initiation complex, causing misreading of the code on the mRNA template and disrupting polysomes.	*E. coli, Enterobacter, Klebsiella, Proteus, Pseudomonas,* and *Serratia* species.
Local		
Neomycin		
Tetracycline	Inhibits protein synthesis by binding to the 30S ribosomal subunit, which interferes with binding of aminoacyl-tRNA.	Mycoplasma, chlamydia, rickettsia, vibrio.
Sulfa drugs		
Sulfonamides	Inhibit folic acid synthesis by competitive inhibition of dihydropteroate synthase.	Gram-positive and -negative organisms, including chlamydia and nocardia.
Trimethoprim	Inhibits folic acid synthesis by inhibition of dihydrofolate reductase.	Used in combination with sulfamethoxazole.
Fluoroquinolones		
Norfloxacin	Inhibits topoisomerase II (DNA gyrase).	Gram-negative organisms, including gonococci, *E. coli, K. pneumoniae, C. jejuni, Enterobacter, Salmonella,* and *Shigella* species.

Drugs for Treating Hypertension

Drug Class	Prototype	Action
Sympathetic nervous system agents		
Central	Clonidine	α_2-agonist; causes decreased sympathetic outflow.
Peripheral	Guanethidine	Uptake by transmitter vesicles in nerve depletes and replaces norepinephrine in neurosecretory vesicles.
	Prazocin	α_1-antagonist.
	Propranolol	β-antagonist.
Central and peripheral	Reserpine	Binds tightly to storage vesicles, which consequently lose their ability to concentrate and store norepinephrine.
Vasodilators		
Arterial	Hydralazine	Unknown.
	Diazoxide	Opens K^+ channels and causes hyperpolarization of smooth muscle.
Arterial and venous	Nitroprusside	Releases NO, which binds to guanylyl cyclase to generate cGMP.
Ca^{++} channel-blockers	Nifedipine	Inhibits voltage-dependent "L-type" Ca^{++} channels.
ACE inhibitors	Captopril	Inhibits conversion of angiotensin I to angiotensin II.
Diuretics		
Thiazides (benzothiadiazides)	Hydrochlorothiazide	Inhibits Na^+ channels in luminal membrane in the proximal segment of the distal tubule.
Loop agents	Furosemide	Inhibits cotransporter of Na^+, K^+, Cl^- in the ascending limb of the loop of Henle.

HIGH-YIELD FACTS

General Principles

Serum concentration vs time
    graphs
    Relationship of drug elimination
      half-time ($t_{1/2}$)
    Apparent volume of distribution
    Drug clearance

Drug distribution
    Henderson-Hasselbalch
      equations
    Diffusion

Partition coefficients

Bioavailability

Log-dose response curves

Anti-Infectives

Cell-wall synthesis inhibitors
    Penicillins
    Cephalosporins
    Monobactams
    Carbapenem
    Vancomycin
    Cycloserine

β-lactamase inhibitors

Protein synthesis inhibitors
    Chloramphenicol
    Tetracyclines
    Macrolides
    Lincosamides
    Aminoglycosides

Folic acid synthesis inhibitors
    Sulfonamides
    Trimethoprim

DNA synthesis inhibitors
    Fluoroquinolones

Antimycobacterials
    Isoniazid
    Rifampin
    Ethambutol
    Pyrizinamide
    Streptomycin

Antileprosy agents

Antifungals
    Amphotericin B
    Flucytosine
    Azoles
    Terbinafine

Antivirals
    Antiherpes agents

Antiretrovirals
    Nucleoside reverse transcriptase
      inhibitors
    Nonnucleoside reverse
      transcriptase inhibitors
    Protease inhibitors
    Amantadine
    Interferons
    Ribavirin

Antiprotozoals

Antihelminthics

Organism	Drug
Pneumococcus	Penicillin G, ampicillin
Pneumococcus (penicillin-resistant)	Fluoroquinolones
Streptococcus	Penicillin G, macrolides (allergic patients)
Staphylococcus (penicillinase-resistant)	Penicillinase-resistant penicillin
Staphylococcus (methicillin-resistant)	Vancomycin
Enterococcus	Penicillin G and gentamycin
Enterococcus (vancomycin-resistant)	Linezolid
Gonococcus	Ceftriaxone, fluoroquinolones
Menigicoccus	Penicillin G, ampicillin, cephtriaxone
Escherichia coli, Proteus, Klebsiella	Second- and third-generation cephalosporin, trimethoprim-sulfamethoxazole, ampicillin, fluoroquinolones
Shigella	Fluoroquinolones
Enterobacter, Serratia	Imipenem, trimethoprim-sulfamethoxazole, fluoroquinolones, pipericillin/tazobactam
Hemophilus	Second- or third-generation cephalosporins, trimethoprim-sulfamethoxazole, fluoroquinolones
Pseudomonas	Cephtazidime, cefepime, imipenem, aztreonam, ciprofloxacin, aminoglycoside, and extended-spectrum penicillin
Bacteroides	Metronidazole, clindamycin
Mycoplasma	Macrolide, tetracycline
Treponema	Penicillin G

Drug	Adverse Drug Reaction
Penicillins	Cross-allergenicity
Cephalosporins	Cross-allergenicity
	Contraindicated in patients with history of anaphylaxis to penicillins
	Disulfiram-like reaction with ethanol
Vancomycin	"Red person" syndrome
Chloramphenicol	"Gray baby syndrome," aplastic anemia
Macrolides	Arrhythmias with coadministration of astemizole

Drug	Adverse Drug Reaction
Clindamycin	Clostridium difficile colitis
Aminoglycosides	Ototoxicity and nephrotoxicity
Tetracycline	Discolored teeth, enamel dysplasia, and bone growth disturbances in children
Sulfa drugs	Cross-allergenicity with other sulfa drugs and with certain diuretics and hypoglycemics
Fluoroquinolones	Tendonitis, Achilles tendon rupture, contraindicated in patients less than 18 years old because of effects on cartilage development
Amphotericin B	Shocklike reaction
Azole antifungals	Arrhythmias with astemizole
Isoniazid	Hepatotoxicity prevented by coadministration of pyridoxine
Ethambutol	Visual disturbances
Pyrazinamide	Nongouty polyarthralgias
Dapsone	Hemolysis in patients with glucose-6-phosphate dehydrogenase deficiency

Antiviral Agent	Adverse Drug Reaction
Zidovudine (AZT)	Anemia
Didanosine (ddI)	Neuropathy, pancreatitis
Stavudine (d4T)	Neuropathy
Abacavir	Hypersensitivity reaction
Efavirenz	Central nervous system toxicity
Protease inhibitors	Hepatotoxicity, hyperlipidemia, nephrolithiasis, lipodystrophy
Acyclovir	Nephropathy
Ganciclovir	Neutropenia
Foscarnet	Renal toxicity
Ribavirin	Anemia
Interferons	Flulike symptoms
Lamivudine	Lactic acidosis
Rimantadine, amantadine	Central nervous system toxicity
Zanamavir	Bronchospasm

Cancer Chemotherapy and Immunology

Cell cycle kinetics

Antimetabolites
  Cell cycle sensitive (CCS)—
    primarily in the S phase
Plant alkaloids
  Vinblastine and vincristine—
    CCS—primarily in the
    M phase
  Ectoposide—CCS—S and early
    G2 phase
  Paclitaxel—spindle poison
Antibiotics
  Bleomycin—CCS—primarily in
    G2 phase
  Doxyrubicin, dactinomycin, and
    mitomycin—cell cycle non-
    sensitive
Alkylating agents and hormones—
    cell cycle nonspecific
    (CCNS)

Cardiovascular and Pulmonary Systems

Drugs used in congestive heart
    failure
  Positive inotropes
  Diuretics
  ACE inhibitors
  PDE inhibitors
  Vasodilators

Antianginals
  Calcium channel blockers
  Nitrates
  β-adrenergic blockers
Antiarrhythmics
  Sodium channel blockers
  β-adrenergic blockers
  Potassium channel blockers
  Calcium channel blockers
  Adenosine
  Digoxin
Antihypertensives
  Diuretics
  Adrenergic receptor blockers
  Vasodilators
  Angiotensin antagonists
Antihyperlipidemics
  Resins
  HMG-CoA reductase inhibitors
  Niacin
  Gemfibrozil
Drugs used in clotting disorders
  Clot reducers
    Anticoagulants
    Antiplatelet agents
    Thrombolytics
  Clot facilitators
    Replacement factors
    Plasminogen inhibitors
Antiasthmatics
  Bronchodilators
  Anti-inflammatories
  Leukotriene antagonists

Drug	Adverse Drug Reaction
Digoxin	Arrythmias, visual aberrations
Nitrates	Tachycardia, headaches, and tolerance
Verapamil	Constipation
β-adrenergic blockers	Bradycardia and asthma
Quinidine and sotalol	Torsades-like arrhythmia
Procainamide	Lupus-like reaction
Amiodarone	Pulmonary fibrosis, thyroid dysfunction, and constipation
Prazosin	First-dose orthostatic hypotension
Clonidine	Rebound hypertension on acute drug cessation
Methyldopa	Positive Coombs test
Guanethidine	Orthostatic hypotension
Reserpine	Depression
Hydralazine	Lupus-like syndrome
Minoxidil	Hirsutism, marked salt and water retention
ACE inhibitors	Dry cough, contraindicated in renal disease
Resins	Bloating
HMG-CoA reductase inhibitors	Severe muscle pain
Niacin	Flushing

Central Nervous System

Antipsychotics
  Phenothiazines
  Thioxanthines
  Butyrophenones
  Heterocyclics
  Antimanics

Adverse Drug Reactions of Antipsychotics

Extrapyramidal effects—haloperidol, fluphenazine

Tardive dyskinesia

Atropine-like effects—thioridizine, chlorpromazine, clozapine

Orthostatic hypotension

Hyperprolactinemia

Amenorrhea-galactorrhea syndrome

Neuroleptic malignant syndrome

Agranulocytosis—clozapine

Nephrogenic diabetes insipidus—lithium

Antidepressants
Monoamine oxidase (MAO) inhibitors
Tricyclics

Heterocyclics
Selective serotonin reuptake
    inhibitors
α_2-adrenergic blockers
Adverse Drug Reactions of Antidepressants
Combination of MAO inhibitors
    and fluoxetine—serotonin
    syndrome
MAO inhibitors and foods containing tyramine—hypertensive
    crisis
Opiates
    Agonists
    Mixed agonists
    Antagonists
Anxiolytics
    Benzodiazepines

Barbiturates
Ethanol
Antiparkinsonians
    Dopamine antagonists
    MAO inhibitors
    Antimuscarinics
Adverse Drug Reactions of Antiparkinsonians
Levodopa, bromocryptine—
    choreoathetosis
Antiepileptics
    Phenytoin
    Carbamazepine
    Valproic acid
    Gabapentin
    Vigabatrin
    Ethosuximide
    Benzodiazepines

Drug	Use
Valproic acid, phenytoin, carbamazine	Grand mal seizures
Ethosuximide, valproic acid	Absence seizures
Valproic acid	Myoclonus
Diazepam, lorazepam	Status epilepticus

Drug	Adverse Drug Reaction
Valproic acid	Neural tube defects
Phenytoin	Nystagmus, gingival hyperplasia, ataxia, hirsutism
Carbamazepine	Diplopia, ataxia
Gabapentin	Movement disorders, behavioral aberrations in children
Vigabatrin	Agitation, confusion, psychosis

Autonomic Nervous System

Location and function of adrenergic
and cholinergic receptors

Cholinergic agents
Direct acting
Nicotinic
Muscarinic
Indirect acting
Organophosphates
Carbamates
Quarternary alcohols
Anticholinergic agents
Antimuscarinic
Antinicotinic

Ganglionic blockers
Neuromuscular blockers
Adrenergic agents
Direct acting
α-adrenergic agonists
β-adrenergic agonists
Indirect acting
Releasers
Reuptake inhibitors
Antiadrenergic agents
α-adrenergic blockers
β-adrenergic blockers

Drug	Use
Edrophonium, pyridostigmine, neostigmine	Myasthenia gravis
Carbachol, pilocarpine, physostigmine, timolol	Glaucoma
Tacrine, donepezil	Alzheimer's disease
Pralidoxime	Organophosphate poisoning antidote
Scopalamime	Motion sickness
Ipratropium	Chronic obstructive pulmonary disease
Albuterol	Asthma
Dopamine	Cardiogenic shock
Dobutamine	Cardiogenic shock and congestive heart failure
Ephedrine, oxymetazoline, phenylephrine	Nasal congestion
Phentolamine, phenoxybenzamine	Pheochromocytoma
Prazosin	Hypertension
Beta blockers	Angina, hypertension, arrhythmias, and myocardial infarction
Epinephrine	Anaphylaxis
Tropicamide	Mydriasis and cycloplegia

Drug	Adverse Drug Reaction
Muscarinics	Nausea, vomiting, diarrhea, salivation, sweating, cutaneous vasodilation, and bronchial constriction
Nicotinics	Convulsions, respiratory paralysis, and hypertension
Cholinesterase inhibitors	Signs of muscarinic and nicotinic toxicities
Antimuscarinics	Hyperthermia due to blockage of sweating mechanisms, decreased salivation and lacrimation, acute-angle-closure glaucoma in the elderly, urinary retention, constipation, blurred vision, delirium, and hallucinations
Antinicotinics	Respiratory paralysis
Adrenergics	Marked increase in blood pressure, tachycardia
α-adrenergic blockers	Orthostatic hypotension, reflex tachycardia
β-adrenergic blockers	Bradycardia, atrioventricular blockade, negative inotropy, bronchiolar constriction, hypoglycemia

Local Control Substances

Histamine antagonists
  H_1
  H_2
Serotonin agonists
  5-H_1
  Serotonin-selective reuptake inhibitors
Serotonin antagonists
  5-HT_2
  5-HT_3
Ergot alkaloids
  CNS
  Uterus
  Vessels

Eicosonoid agonists
  Prostaglandins
  Prostacyclins
  Thromboxanes
  Leukotrienes
Eicosonoid antagonists
  Corticosteroids
  Nonsteroidal anti-inflammatory drugs (NSAIDs)
  Leukotriene antagonists

Drug	Use
Histamine antagonists	
H_1	Allergies
H_2	Acid-peptic disease
Serotonin agonists	
Sumatriptan	Acute migraine and cluster headaches
Serotonin antagonists	
Ketanserin, cyproheptadine, and phenoxybenzamine	Carcinoid tumors
Ondansetron	Postoperative vomiting and vomiting associated with cancer chemotherapy
Ergot alkaloids	
Ergotamine	Acute migraine headache
Methysergide and ergonovine	Prophylactic use for migraine headaches
Ergonovine and ergotamine	Reduction of postpartum bleeding
Bromocryptine and pergolide	Reduction of prolactin secretion
Eicosanoid agonists	
Misoprostol	Abortifacient, prevention of ulcers in combination with NSAIDs therapy
PGE_1	Maintain patency of ductus arteriosus
Alprostadil	Erectile dysfunction
Corticosteroids	Inhibition of arachidonic acid production
NSAIDs	Closure of patent ductus arteriosus
Indomethacin	Asthma
Leukotriene antagonists	

Drug	Adverse Drug Reaction
Histamine receptor antagonists	
H_1	Drowsiness
H_2-cimetidine	Inhibitor of drug-metabolizing enzymes
Serotonin antagonists	
Ketanserin	α and H_1 antagonism
Ondansetron	Diarrhea and headache
Ergot alkaloids	Ischemia and gangrene, fibroplasia of connective tissue, uterine contractions, and hallucinations

Renal System

Diuretics effecting salt and water
  excretion
  Osmotic
  Carbonic anhydrase inhibitors
  Loop diuretics
  Thiazides

Potassium-sparing diuretics
Drugs effecting water excretion
  Osmotic
  ADH agonists
  ADH antagonists

Drug	Use
Loop diuretics	Congestive heart failure and pulmonary edema, ascites
Thiazides	Hypertension, congestive heart failure, renal calcium stones
Osmotics	Increasing urine flow, decreasing intracranial pressure
Potassium-sparing diuretics	Diminishing potassium wasting from other diuretics
ADH	Pituitary diabetes insipidus

Drug	Adverse Drug Reaction
Loop diuretics	Hypokalemia, ototoxicity
Thiazides	Hypokalemia, hyperglycemia, hyperuricemia, hyperlipidemia
Potassium-sparing diuretics	Hyperkalemia
Spironolactone	Gynecomastia and antiandrogenic effects
ADH	Hyponatremia

Gastrointestinal System and Nutrition

Gastrointestinal tract ulcers
  Antacids
  Polymers (sucralfate)
  Proton pump inhibitors
  Antibiotics

Gastrointestinal motility
  promotors
  Antiemetics
  H_2 antagonists
  Phenothiazines
  5-HT inhibitors

Pancreatic replacement enzymes
Laxatives
Irritants
Bulk formers

Stool softeners
Lubricants
Sulfasalazine
Antidiarrheals

Drug	Use
Ondansetron	Antiemetic in cancer chemotherapy
Omeprazole	Zollinger-Ellison syndrome

Endocrine System

Androgens
  Testosterone

Antiandrogens
  GnRH analogs
  Steroid synthesis inhibitors
  5α reductase inhibitors
  Testosterone receptor inhibitors

Estrogens

Progesterones

Corticosteroids
  Glucocorticoids
  Mineralocorticoids

Corticosteroid antagonists

Receptor antagonists

Synthetic inhibitors

Thyroid hormones
  Thyroxine
  Triiodothyronine

Antithyroid hormones
  Thioamides
  Iodide

Radioactive iodide
Ipodate

Antidiabetics
  Insulin
  Oral hypoglycemics
    Sulfonylureas
    Biguanides
    Thiazolidinediones
    Acarbose

Hyperglycemics

Bone mineral metabolism agents
  Parathyroid hormone
  Vitamin D
  Calcitonin—Paget's disease and hypercalcemia
  Estrogens
  Glucocorticoids
  Biphosphonates—postmenopausal osteoporosis
  Fluoride
  Plicamycin—Paget's disease

Drug	Adverse Drug Reaction
Androgens	Masculinizing effects
Estrogens	Breakthrough bleeding and breast tenderness
Thyroid hormones	Thyrotoxicosis
Glucocorticoids	Adrenal suppression, salt retention, diabetes, osteoporosis
Insulin	Hypoglycemia
Sulfonylureas	Hypoglycemia
Biguanides	Diarrhea, lactic acidosis in renal or hepatic insufficiency and anoxic states
Thiazolidinediones	Possible hepatotoxicity
Etidronate	Esophageal irritation
Fluoride	Ectopic bone formation, exostosis
Vitamin D	Nephrocalcinosis

Toxicology

Air pollutants
  Carbon monoxide
  Sulfur dioxide
  Nitrogen oxides
  Ozone
Solvents
  Halogenated hydrocarbons
  Aromatic hydrocarbons
Insecticides
  Chlorinated hydrocarbons
  Cholinesterase inhibitors
  Botanical insecticides

Herbicides
Environmental pollutants
  Dioxins
  Polychlorinated biphenyls
Heavy metals
  Lead
  Arsenic
  Mercury
  Iron

Toxin	Treatment
Carbon dioxide	Removal from exposure and administer oxygen
Sulfur dioxide	Removal from exposure
Aliphatic hydrocarbons	Removal from exposure
Aromatic hydrocarbons	Removal from exposure
Cholinesterase inhibitors	Atropine, pralidoxime
Paraquat	Gastric lavage and dialysis
Lead	Dimercaprol, penicillamine
Arsenic	Dimercaprol, penicillamine
Mercury	Dimercaprol (elemental), penicillamine, dimercaprol (inorganic salts)
Iron	Deferoxamine

General Principles

Drug-receptor interactions
Dose-response relationships
Molecular models of receptors and
  signal transduction mechanisms
Biotransformation
Pharmacokinetics
Pharmacodynamics

Dosage regimens and pharmaco-
  kinetic profiles
Factors affecting drug dosage
Development of new drugs
Regulation by the Food and Drug
  Administration

Questions

DIRECTIONS: Each item below contains a question or incomplete statement followed by suggested responses. Select the **one best** response to each question.

1. Of the many types of data plots that are used to help explain the pharmacodynamics of drugs, which plot is very useful for determining the total number of receptors and the affinity of a drug for those receptors in a tissue or membrane?

a. Graded dose-response curve
b. Quantal dose-response curve
c. Scatchard plot
d. Double-reciprocal plot
e. Michaelis-Menten plot

2. Which route of administration is most likely to subject a drug to a first-pass effect?

a. Intravenous
b. Inhalational
c. Oral
d. Sublingual (SL)
e. Intramuscular

3. Two drugs may act on the same tissue or organ through independent receptors, resulting in effects in opposite directions. This is known as

a. Physiologic antagonism
b. Chemical antagonism
c. Competitive antagonism
d. Irreversible antagonism
e. Dispositional antagonism

Questions 4–7

A new aminoglycoside antibiotic (5 mg/kg) was infused intravenously over 30 min to a 70-kg volunteer. The plasma concentrations of the drug were measured at various times after the end of the infusion, as recorded in the table and shown in the figure below.

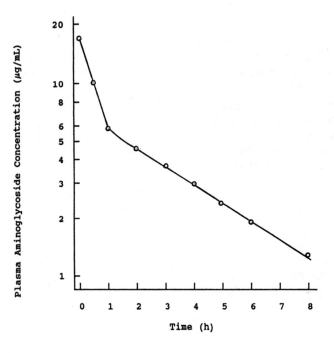

Time After Dosing Stopped (h)	Plasma Aminoglycoside Concentration (mg/mL)
0.0	18.0
0.5	10.0
1.0	5.8
2.0	4.6
3.0	3.7
4.0	3.0
5.0	2.4
6.0	1.9
8.0	1.3

4. The elimination half-life ($t_{1/2}$) of the aminoglycoside in this patient was approximately

a. 0.6 h
b. 1.2 h
c. 2.1 h
d. 3.1 h
e. 4.2 h

5. The elimination rate constant (k_e) of the aminoglycoside in this patient was approximately

a. 0.15 h^{-1}
b. 0.22 h^{-1}
c. 0.33 h^{-1}
d. 0.60 h^{-1}
e. 1.13 h^{-1}

6. The apparent volume of distribution (V_d) of the drug in this patient was approximately

a. 0.62 L
b. 19 L
c. 50 L
d. 110 L
e. 350 L

7. The total body clearance (CL_{total}) of the drug in this patient was approximately

a. 11 L/h
b. 23 L/h
c. 35 L/h
d. 47 L/h
e. 65 L/h

8. If a drug is repeatedly administered at dosing intervals that are equal to its elimination half-life, the number of doses required for the plasma concentration of the drug to reach the steady state is

a. 2 to 3
b. 4 to 5
c. 6 to 7
d. 8 to 9
e. 10 or more

9. The pharmacokinetic value that most reliably reflects the amount of drug reaching the target tissue after oral administration is the

a. Peak blood concentration
b. Time to peak blood concentration
c. Product of the V_d and the first-order rate constant
d. V_d
e. Area under the blood concentration-time curve (AUC)

10. It was determined that 95% of an oral 80-mg dose of verapamil was absorbed in a 70-kg test subject. However, because of extensive biotransformation during its first pass through the portal circulation, the bioavailability of verapamil was only 25%. Assuming a liver blood flow of 1500 mL/min, the hepatic clearance of verapamil in this situation was

a. 60 mL/min
b. 375 mL/min
c. 740 mL/min
d. 1110 mL/min
e. 1425 mL/min

11. Drug products have many types of names. Of the following types of names that are applied to drugs, the one that is the official name and refers only to that drug and not to a particular product is the

a. Generic name
b. Trade name
c. Brand name
d. Chemical name
e. Proprietary name

12. Which of the following is classified as belonging to the tyrosine kinase family of receptors?

a. GABA$_A$ receptor
b. β-adrenergic receptor
c. Insulin receptor
d. Nicotinic II receptor
e. Hydrocortisone receptor

13. Identical doses of a capsule preparation (X) and a tablet preparation (Y) of the same drug were compared on a blood concentration-time plot with respect to peak concentration, time to peak concentration, and AUC after oral administration as shown in the figure below. This comparison was made to determine which of the following?

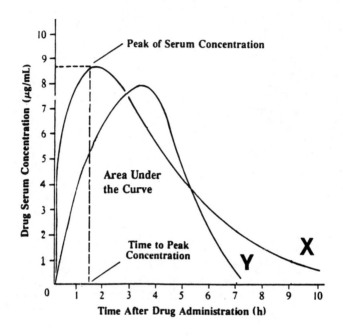

a. Potency
b. Extent of plasma protein binding
c. Bioequivalence
d. Therapeutic effectiveness
e. None of the above

14. Of the following characteristics, which is unlikely to be associated with the process of facilitated diffusion of drugs?

a. The transport mechanism becomes saturated at high drug concentrations
b. The process is selective for certain ionic or structural configurations of the drug
c. If two compounds are transported by the same mechanism, one will competitively inhibit the transport of the other
d. The drug crosses the membrane against a concentration gradient and the process requires cellular energy
e. The transport process can be inhibited noncompetitively by substances that interfere with cellular metabolism

15. In comparing the following possible routes, which is associated with the excretion of quantitatively small amounts of drugs or their metabolic derivatives?

a. Biliary tract
b. Kidneys
c. Lungs
d. Feces
e. Milk

16. Of the following, which is a phase II biotransformation reaction?

a. Sulfoxide formation
b. Nitro reduction
c. Ester hydrolysis
d. Sulfate conjugation
e. Deamination

17. Which of the following is unlikely to be associated with oral drug administration of an enteric-coated dosage form?

a. Irritation to the gastric mucosa with nausea and vomiting
b. Destruction of the drug by gastric acid or digestive enzymes
c. Unpleasant taste of the drug
d. Formation of nonabsorbable drug-food complexes
e. Variability in absorption caused by fluctuations in gastric emptying time

18. Of the following, which is unlikely to be associated with receptors bound to plasma membranes, their interaction with ligands, and the biologic response to this interaction?

a. Structurally, these receptors have hydrophobic amino acid domains, which are in contact with the membrane, and hydrophilic regions, which extend into the extracellular fluid and the cytoplasm
b. Chemical interactions of ligands with these receptors may involve the formation of many types of bonds, including ionic, hydrogen, van der Waals', and covalent
c. Ligand-receptor interactions are often stereospecific (i.e., one stereoisomer is usually more potent than the other)
d. In some cases, a ligand that acts as an agonist at membrane-bound receptors increases the activity of an intracellular second messenger
e. Activation of membrane-bound receptors and subsequent intracellular events elicit a biologic response through the transcription of DNA

19. Of the following, which is unlikely to be associated with the binding of drugs to plasma proteins?

a. Acidic drugs generally bind to plasma albumin; basic drugs preferentially bind to α_1-acidic glycoprotein
b. Plasma protein binding is a reversible process
c. Binding sites on plasma proteins are nonselective, and drugs with similar physicochemical characteristics compete for these limited sites
d. The fraction of the drug in the plasma that is bound is inactive and generally unavailable for systemic distribution
e. Plasma protein binding generally limits renal tubular secretion and biotransformation

20. Of the following, which is unlikely to be associated with drug distribution into and out of the central nervous system (CNS)?

a. The blood-brain barrier, which involves drug movement through glial cell membranes as well as capillary membranes, is the main hindrance to drug distribution to the CNS
b. Most drugs enter the CNS by simple diffusion at rates that are proportional to the lipid solubility of the nonionized form of the drug
c. Receptor-mediated transport allows certain peptides to gain access to the brain
d. Strongly ionized drugs freely enter the CNS through carrier-mediated transport systems
e. Some drugs leave the CNS by passing from the cerebrospinal fluid into the dural blood sinuses through the arachnoid villi

21. The greater proportion of the dose of a drug administered orally will be absorbed in the small intestine. However, on the assumption that passive transport of the nonionized form of a drug determines its rate of absorption, which of the following compounds will be absorbed to the least extent in the stomach?

a. Ampicillin ($pK_a = 2.5$)
b. Aspirin ($pK_a = 3.0$)
c. Warfarin ($pK_a = 5.0$)
d. Phenobarbital ($pK_a = 7.4$)
e. Propranolol ($pK_a = 9.4$)

DIRECTIONS: Each group of questions below consists of lettered options followed by a set of numbered items. For each numbered item, select the **one** lettered option with which it is **most** closely associated. Each lettered option may be used once, more than once, or not at all.

Questions 22–24

For each type of drug interaction below, select the pair of substances that illustrates it with a *reduction* in drug effectiveness:

a. Tetracycline and milk
b. Amobarbital and secobarbital
c. Isoproterenol and propranolol
d. Soap and benzalkonium chloride
e. Sulfamethoxazole and trimethoprim

22. Therapeutic interaction

23. Physical interaction

24. Chemical interaction

Questions 25–27

For each description of a drug response below, choose the term with which it is most likely to be associated:

a. Supersensitivity
b. Tachyphylaxis
c. Tolerance
d. Hyposensitivity
e. Anaphylaxis

25. Immunologically mediated reaction to drug observed soon after administration

26. A rapid reduction in the effect of a given dose of a drug after only one or two doses

27. Hyperreactivity to a drug seen as a result of denervation

Questions 28–30

For each component of a time-action curve listed below, choose the lettered interval (shown on the diagram) with which it is most closely associated:

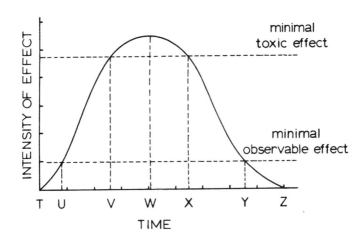

a. T to U
b. T to V
c. T to W
d. T to Z
e. U to V
f. U to W
g. U to X
h. U to Y
i. V to X
j. X to Y

28. Time to peak effect

29. Time to onset of action

30. Duration of action

Questions 31–33

For each description below, select the transmembranal transport mechanism it best defines:

a. Filtration
b. Simple diffusion
c. Facilitated diffusion
d. Active transport
e. Endocytosis

31. Lipid-soluble drugs cross the membrane at a rate proportional to the concentration gradient across the membrane and the lipid:water partition coefficient of the drug

32. Bulk flow of water through membrane pores, resulting from osmotic differences across the membrane, transports drug molecules that fit through the membrane pores

33. After binding to a proteinaceous membrane carrier, drugs are carried across the membrane (with the expenditure of cellular energy), where they are released

Questions 34–36

Lipid-soluble xenobiotics are commonly biotransformed by oxidation in the drug-metabolizing microsomal system (DMMS). For each description below, choose the component of the microsomal mixed-function oxidase system with which it is most closely associated:

a. Nicotinamide adenine dinucleotide phosphate (NADPH)
b. Cytochrome a
c. Adenosine triphosphate (ATP)
d. NADPH–cytochrome P450 reductase
e. Monoamine oxidase (MAO)
f. Cyclooxygenase
g. Cytochrome P450

34. A group of iron (Fe)-containing isoenzymes that activate molecular oxygen to a form that is capable of interacting with organic substrates

35. The component that provides reducing equivalents for the enzyme system

36. A flavoprotein that accepts reducing equivalents and transfers them to the catalytic enzyme

General Principles

Answers

1. The answer is c. *(Hardman, pp 37–38.)* Based on the concept that, for most situations, the association of a drug with its receptor is reversible, the following reaction applies:

$$D + R \underset{k_2}{\overset{k_1}{\rightleftarrows}} DR \rightarrow Effect$$

where D is the concentration of free drug, R is the concentration of receptors, DR is the concentration of drug bound to its receptors, and K_D (equal to k_2/k_1) is the equilibrium dissociation constant. The affinity of a drug for its receptor is estimated from the dissociation constant in that its reciprocal, $1/K_D$, is the affinity constant. All of the plots listed in the question can be used to quantitate some aspect of drug action. For example, K_D can be determined from the Michaelis-Menten relationship, graded dose-response curves, and the Scatchard plot. However, only the Scatchard plot can be

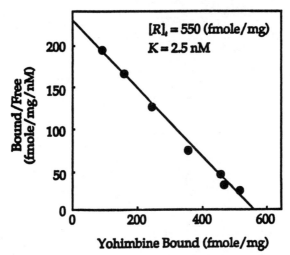

(From Neubig RR, Gantros RD, and Brasier RS: Mol Pharmacol *28:475–486, 1985, with permission.)*

used to determine the total number of receptors in a tissue or membrane. This is accomplished by measuring the binding of a radioactively labeled drug to a membrane or tissue preparation in vitro. A Scatchard plot of the binding of ^{3}H-yohimbine to α_2-adrenergic receptors on human platelet membranes is shown on the previous page as an example. A plot of DR/D (bound/free drug) vs. DR (bound drug) yields a slope of $1/K_D$ (the affinity constant) and an x intercept of R (total number of receptors).

Scatchard analysis is very useful in certain therapeutic situations. For example, this type of analysis is used to determine the number of estrogen receptors present in a biopsy of breast tissue prior to developing a drug treatment regimen for breast cancer in a patient.

2. The answer is c. *(Hardman, p 5.)* The first-pass effect is commonly considered to involve the biotransformation of a drug during its first passage through the portal circulation of the liver. Drugs that are administered orally and rectally enter the portal circulation of the liver and can be biotransformed by this organ prior to reaching the systemic circulation. Therefore, drugs with a high first-pass effect are highly biotransformed quickly, which reduces the oral bioavailability and the systemic blood concentrations of the compounds. Administration by the intravenous, intramuscular, and sublingual routes allows the drug to attain concentrations in the systemic circulation and to be distributed throughout the body prior to hepatic metabolism. In most cases, drugs administered by inhalation are not subjected to a significant first-pass effect unless the respiratory tissue is a major site for the drug's biotransformation.

3. The answer is a. *(Hardman, p 68.)* Physiologic, or *functional, antagonism* occurs when two drugs produce opposite effects on the same physiologic function, often by interacting with different types of receptors. A practical example of this is the use of epinephrine as a bronchodilator to counteract the bronchoconstriction that occurs following histamine release from mast cells in the respiratory tract during a severe allergic reaction. Histamine constricts the bronchioles by stimulating histamine H_1 receptors in the tissue; epinephrine relaxes this tissue through its agonistic activity on β_2-adrenergic receptors.

Chemical antagonism results when two drugs combine with each other chemically and the activity of one or both is blocked. For example, dimercaprol chelates lead and reduces the toxicity of this heavy metal. Competitive antagonism, or inactivation, occurs when two compounds compete for the same receptor site; this is a reversible interaction. Thus, atropine blocks the effects of acetylcholine on the heart by competing with the neurotransmitter for binding to cardiac muscarinic receptors. Irreversible antagonism generally results from the binding of an antagonist to the same receptor site as the agonist by covalent interaction or by a very slowly dissociating noncovalent interaction. An example of this antagonism is the blockade produced by phenoxybenzamine on α-adrenergic receptors, resulting in a long-lasting reduction in the activity of norepinephrine.

Dispositional antagonism occurs when one drug alters the pharmacokinetics (absorption, distribution, biotransformation, or excretion) of a second drug so that less of the active compound reaches the target tissue. For example, phenobarbital induces the biotransformation of warfarin, reducing its anticoagulant activity.

4. The answer is d. *(Katzung, pp 35–41.)* The figure that accompanies the question shows an elimination pattern with two distinct components, which typifies a two-compartment model. The upper portion of the line represents the α phase, which is the distribution of the drug from the tissues that receive high rates of blood flow [the central compartment (e.g., the brain, heart, kidney, and lungs)] to the tissues with lower rates of blood flow [the peripheral compartment (e.g., skeletal muscle, adipose tissue, and bone)]. Once distribution to all tissue is complete, equilibrium occurs throughout the body. The elimination of the drug from the body (the β phase) is represented by the lower linear portion of the line; this part of the line is used to determine the elimination half-life of the drug.

At 2 h after dosing, the plasma concentration was 4.6 mg/mL; at 5 h, the concentration was 2.4 mg/mL. Therefore, the plasma concentration of this aminoglycoside decreased to one-half in approximately 3 h—its half-life. In addition, drug elimination usually occurs according to first-order kinetics (i.e., a linear relationship is obtained when the drug concentration is plotted on a logarithmic scale vs. time on an arithmetic scale (a semilogarithmic plot)].

5. The answer is b. *(Katzung, p 40.)* The fraction change in drug concentration per unit of time for any first-order process is expressed by k_e. This constant is related to the half-life $(t_{1/2})$ by the equation $k_e t_{1/2} = 0.693$. The units of k_e are time^{-1}, while the $t_{1/2}$ is expressed in units of time. By substitution of the appropriate value for half-life estimated from the data from the graph or table accompanying the question (the β phase) into the preceding equation, rearranged to solve for k_e, the answer is calculated as follows:

$$k_e = \frac{0.693}{t_{1/2}} = \frac{0.693}{3.0\ h} = 0.23\ h^{-1}$$

The problem can also be solved mathematically:

$$\log (A) = \log (A_0) - \frac{k_e}{2.303}\ t$$

where (A_0) is the initial drug concentration, (A) is the final drug concentration, t is the time interval between the two values, and k_e is the elimination rate constant. For example, by solving for k_e using the plasma concentration values at 2 and 5 h,

$$\log (2.4\ mg/mL) = \log (4.6\ mg/mL) - \frac{k_e}{2.303}\ 3\ h$$

k_e will equal $0.22\ h^{-1}$.

6. The answer is c. *(Katzung, p 35.)* The apparent V_d is defined as the volume of fluid into which a drug appears to distribute with a concentration equal to that of plasma, or the volume of fluid necessary to dissolve the drug and yield the same concentration as that found in plasma. By convention, the value of the plasma concentration at zero time is used. In this problem, a hypothetical plasma concentration of the drug at zero time (7 mg/mL) can be estimated by extrapolating the linear portion of the elimination curve (the β phase) back to zero time. Therefore, the apparent V_d is calculated by

$$V_d = \frac{\text{Total amount of drug in the body}}{\text{Drug concentration in plasma at zero time}}$$

Since the total amount of drug in the body is the intravenous dose, 350 mg (i.e., 5 mg/kg × 70 kg), and the estimated plasma concentration at zero time is 7 mg/mL, substitution of these numbers in the equation yields the apparent V_d:

$$V_d = \frac{350\ mg}{7\ mg/mL} = 50\ L$$

7. The answer is a. *(Katzung, pp 36–40.)* Clearance by an organ is defined as the apparent volume of a biologic fluid from which a drug is removed by elimination processes per unit of time. The total body clearance (CL_{total}) is defined as the sum of clearances of all the organs and tissues that eliminate a drug. CL_{total} is influenced by the apparent V_d and k_e. The more rapidly a drug is cleared, the greater is the value of CL_{total}. Therefore, for the new aminoglycoside in this patient,

$$CL_{total} = V_d k_e = (50 \text{ l.}) (0.22 \text{ h}^{-1}) = 11 \text{ L/h}$$

8. The answer is b. *(Hardman, p 23.)* When a drug is administered in multiple doses and each dose is given prior to the complete elimination of the previous dose, the mean plasma concentration (C) of the drug during each dose interval rises as shown in the following figure:

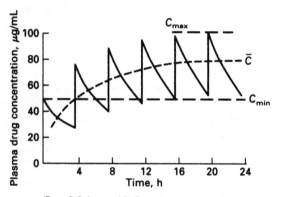

(From DiPalma and DiGregorio, with permission.)

The plasma concentration will continue to rise until it reaches a plateau, or steady state. At this time, the plasma concentration will fluctuate between a maximum (C_{max}) and a minimum (C_{min}) level, but, more important, the amount of drug eliminated per dose interval will equal the amount of drug absorbed per dose. When a drug is given at a dosing interval that is equal to its elimination half-life, it will reach 50% of its steady-state plasma concentration after one half-life, 75% after two half-lives, 87.5% after three, 93.75% after four, and 96.87% after five. Thus, from a practical viewpoint, regardless of the magnitude of the dose or the half-life, the steady state will be achieved in four to five half-lives.

9. The answer is e. (*Hardman, p 21.*) The fraction of a drug dose absorbed after oral administration is affected by a wide variety of factors that can strongly influence the peak blood levels and the time to peak blood concentration. The V_d and the total body clearance ($V_d \times$ first-order k_e) also are important in determining the amount of drug that reaches the target tissue. Only the area under the blood concentration-time curve, however, reflects absorption, distribution, metabolism, and excretion factors; it is the most reliable and popular method of evaluating bioavailability.

10. The answer is d. (*Hardman, pp 4–9. Katzung, pp 41–43.*) *Bioavailability* is defined as the fraction or percentage of a drug that becomes available to the systemic circulation following administration by any route. This takes into consideration that not all of an orally administered drug is absorbed and that a drug can be removed from the plasma and biotransformed by the liver during its initial passage through the portal circulation. A bioavailability of 25% indicates that only 20 mg of the 80-mg dose (i.e., 80 mg $\times$ 0.25 = 20 mg) reached the systemic circulation. Organ clearance can be determined by knowing the blood flow through the organ (Q) and the extraction ratio (ER) for the drug by the organ, according to the equation

$$CL_{organ} = Q \times ER$$

The extraction ratio is dependent upon the amounts of drug entering (C_i) and exiting (C_o) the organ:

$$ER = \frac{C_i \times C_o}{C_i}$$

In this problem, the amount of verapamil entering the liver was 76 mg (80 mg $\times$ 0.95) and the amount leaving was 20 mg. Therefore,

$$ER = \frac{76 \text{ mg} - 20 \text{ mg}}{76 \text{ mg}} = 0.74$$

$$CL_{liver} = (1500 \text{ mL/min}) (0.74) = 1110 \text{ mL/min}$$

11. The answer is a. *(Hardman, pp 55–57.)* When a new chemical entity is first synthesized by a pharmaceutical company, it is given a *chemical name* (e.g., acetylsalicylic acid). During the process of investigation of the usefulness of the new chemical as a drug, it is given a *generic name* by the United States Adopted Names (USAN) Council, which negotiates with the pharmaceutical manufacturer in the choice of a meaningful and distinctive generic name for the new drug. This name will be the established, official name that can only be applied to that one unique drug compound (e.g., aspirin). The *trade name* (or *brand name*, or *proprietary name*) is a registered name given to the product by the pharmaceutical company that is manufacturing or distributing the drug and identifies a particular product containing that drug (e.g., Ecotrin). Thus, acetylsalicylic acid, aspirin, and Ecotrin, for example, all refer to the same therapeutic drug entity; however, only aspirin is the official generic name.

12. The answer is c. *(Hardman, pp 31–34.)* There are four major classes of receptors: (1) ion channel receptors, (2) receptors coupled to G proteins, (3) receptors with tyrosine-specific kinase activity, and (4) nuclear receptors. In most cases, drugs that act via receptors do so by binding to extracellular receptors that transduce the information intracellularly by a variety of mechanisms. Activated ion channel receptors enhance the influx of extracellular ions into the cell; for example, the nicotinic-II cholinergic receptor selectively opens a channel for sodium ions and the $GABA_A$ receptor functions as an ionophore for chloride ions. Receptors coupled to guanine nucleotide-binding proteins (G proteins) act either by opening an ion channel or by stimulating or inhibiting specific enzymes (e.g., β-adrenergic receptor stimulation leads to an increase in cellular adenylate cyclase activity). When stimulated, receptors with tyrosine-specific protein kinase activity activate this enzyme to enhance the transport of ions and nutrients across the cell membrane; for example, insulin receptors function in this manner and increase glucose transport into insulin-dependent tissues. Steroid hormone receptors are different from all the above in that they are associated with the nucleus of the cell and are activated by steroid hormones (e.g., hydrocortisone) that penetrate into target cells. These receptors interact with DNA to enhance genetic transcription.

13. The answer is c. *(Katzung, pp 41–43.)* Drug absorption can vary significantly depending upon the product formulation used and the route of administration. The degree to which a drug achieves a particular concentration in the blood following administration by a route other than intravenous injection is a measure of its efficiency of absorption—its *bioavailability*. When a drug is produced by different processes (e.g., at different manufacturing sites or using different manufacturing or production techniques) or in a different dosage form (e.g., capsule, tablet, suspension) and contains the same amount of active ingredient and is to be used for the same therapeutic purpose, the extent to which the bioavailability of one dosage form differs from that of another must be evaluated. In the body, these dosage forms should produce similar blood or plasma concentration-time curves. The comparison of the bioavailability of two such dosage forms is called *bioequivalence.*

The bioequivalence of different preparations is assessed by an evaluation of three parameters: (1) the peak height concentration achieved by the drug in the dosage form, (2) the time to reach the peak concentration of the drug, and (3) the area under the concentration-time curve. The ascending limb of the curve is considered to be a general reflection of the rate of drug absorption from the dosage form. The descending limb of the concentration-time curve is a general indication of the rate of elimination of the drug from the body.

None of the other choices in the question (i.e., potency, effectiveness, or plasma protein binding) can be evaluated using this type of comparison.

14. The answer is d. *(Hardman, pp 3–4.)* Drugs can be transferred across biologic membranes by passive processes (i.e., filtration and simple diffusion) and by specialized processes (i.e., active transport, facilitated diffusion, and pinocytosis). Active transport is a carrier-mediated process that shows all of the characteristics listed in the question. Facilitated diffusion is similar to active transport except that the drug is not transported against a concentration gradient and no energy is required for this carrier-mediated system to function. Pinocytosis usually involves transport of proteins and macromolecules by a complex process in which a cell engulfs the compound within a membrane-bound vesicle.

15. The answer is e. *(Hardman, pp 16–17.)* The amounts of drugs that are excreted in milk are small compared with those that are excreted by other routes, but drugs in milk may have significant, undesired pharmacologic effects on breast-fed infants. The principal route of excretion of the products of a given drug varies with the drug. Some drugs are predominantly excreted by the kidneys, whereas others leave the body in the bile and feces. Inhalation anesthetic agents are eliminated by the lungs. The path of excretion may affect the clinical choice of a drug, as is the case with renal failure or hepatic insufficiency.

16. The answer is d. (*Hardman, pp 11–16.*) Biotransformation reactions involving the oxidation, reduction, or hydrolysis of a drug are classified as phase I (or nonsynthetic) reactions; these chemical reactions may result in either the activation or inactivation of a pharmacologic agent. There are many types of these reactions; oxidations are the most numerous. Phase II (or synthetic) reactions, which almost always result in the formation of an inactive product, involve conjugation of the drug (or its derivative) with an amino acid, carbohydrate, acetate, or sulfate. The conjugated form(s) of the drug or its derivatives may be more easily excreted than the parent compound.

17. The answer is e. (*Katzung, p 602.*) Tasteless enteric-coated tablets and capsules are formulated to resist the acidic pH found in the stomach. Once the preparation has passed into the intestine, the coating dissolves in the alkaline milieu and releases the drug. Therefore, gastric irritation, drug destruction by gastric acid, and the forming of complexes of the drug with food constituents will be avoided.

18. The answer is e. (*Hardman, pp 31–34.*) Based upon the molecular mechanisms with which receptors transduce signals, four major classes of receptors have been identified: (1) ion channel receptors, (2) receptors that interact with G proteins, (3) receptors with tyrosine kinase activity, and (4) nuclear receptors. The first three types of receptors are complex membrane-bound proteins with hydrophilic regions located within the lipoid cell membrane and hydrophilic portions found protruding into the cytoplasm of the cell and the extracellular milieu; when activated, all of these receptors transmit (or transduce) information presented at the extracellular surface into ionic or biochemical signals within the cell (i.e., second messengers). Nuclear receptors are found in the nucleus of the cell, not bound to plasma membranes. In addition, these receptors do not transduce information by second-messenger systems; rather, they bind to nuclear chromatin and elicit a biologic response through the transcription of DNA and alterations in the formation of cellular proteins. Ligand binding to all types of receptors may involve the formation of ionic, hydrogen, hydrophobic, van der Waals', and covalent bonds. In most cases, ligand-receptor interactions are stereospecific; for example, natural (−)-epinephrine is 1000 times more potent than (+)-epinephrine.

19. The answer is e. (*Hardman, pp 10–11.*) Because only the free (unbound) fraction of a drug can cross biologic membranes, binding to plasma proteins limits a drug's concentration in tissues and, therefore, decreases the apparent V_d of the drug. Plasma protein binding will also reduce glomerular filtration of the drug because this process is highly dependent on the free drug fraction. Renal tubular secretion and biotransformation of drugs are generally not limited by plasma protein binding because these processes reduce the free drug concentration in the plasma. If a drug is avidly transported through the tubule by the secretion process or is rapidly biotransformed, the rates of these processes may exceed the rate of dissociation of the drug-protein complex (in order to restore the free:bound drug ratio in plasma) and, thus, become the rate-limiting factor for drug elimination. This assumes that equilibrium conditions exist and that other influences (e.g., changes in pH or the presence of other drugs) do not occur.

20. The answer is d. (*Hardman, pp 9–10.*) Drugs can enter the brain from the circulation by passing through the blood-brain barrier. This boundary consists of several membranes, including those of the capillary wall, the glial cells closely surrounding the capillary, and the neuron. In most cases, lipid-soluble drugs diffuse through these membranes at rates that are related to their lipid-to-water partition coefficients. Therefore, the greater the lipid solubility of the nonionized fraction of a weak acid or base, the more freely permeable the drug is to the brain. Some drugs enter the CNS through specific carrier-mediated or receptor-mediated transport processes. Carrier-mediated systems appear to be involved predominantly in the transport of a variety of nutrients through the blood-brain barrier; however, the thyroid hormone 3,5,3′-triiodothyronine and drugs such as levodopa and methyldopa, which are structural derivatives of phenylalanine, cross the blood-brain barrier via carrier-mediated transport. Receptor-mediated transport functions to permit a peptide (e.g., insulin) to enter the CNS; therefore, some peptide-like drugs are believed to gain access to the brain by this mechanism. Regardless of the process by which drugs can enter the CNS, strongly ionized drugs (e.g., quaternary amines) are unable to enter the CNS from the blood.

The exit of drugs from the CNS can involve (1) diffusion across the blood-brain barrier in the reverse direction at rates determined by the lipid solubility and degree of ionization of the drug, (2) drainage from the cerebrospinal fluid (CSF) into the dural blood sinuses by flowing through the wide channels of the arachnoid villi, and (3) active transport of certain organic anions and cations from the CSF to blood across the choroid plexuses.

21. The answer is e. *(Hardman, pp 4–5. Katzung, pp 5–7.)* Weak acids and weak bases are dissociated into nonionized and ionized forms, depending upon the pK_a of the molecule and the pH of the environment. The nonionized form of a drug passes through cellular membranes more easily than the ionized form because it is more lipid soluble. Thus, the rate of passive transport varies with the proportion of the drug that is nonionized. When the pH of the environment in which a weak acid or weak base drug is contained is equal to the pK_a, the drug is 50% dissociated. Weak acids (e.g., salicylates, barbiturates) are more readily absorbed from the stomach than from other regions of the alimentary canal because a large percentage of these weak acids are in the nonionized state. The magnitude of this effect can be estimated by applying the Henderson-Hasselbalch equation:

$$\log\left(\frac{\text{Protonated form}}{\text{Unprotonated form}}\right) = pK_a - pH$$

At an acidic pH of about 3, of the drugs in question, all are weak acids except propranolol; therefore, propranolol has the greatest percentage of its molecules in the ionized form in the stomach. The higher the value of the pK_a, the less ionized these substances are in the stomach.

22–24. The answers are 22-c, 23-d, 24-a. *(Katzung, pp 4–5, 1122–1123.)* A therapeutic drug interaction is one that reduces drug effectiveness results when two drugs with opposing pharmacologic effects are administered. For example, isoproterenol, a β-adrenergic stimulator, will antagonize the effect of propranolol, a β-adrenergic blocking agent. The combined use of amobarbital and secobarbital, both barbiturate sedative-hypnotics, represents a drug interaction that causes an additive (enhanced) pharmacologic response (i.e., depression of the CNS). The combination of the antimicrobials sulfamethoxazole and trimethoprim is an example of a very useful drug interaction in which one drug potentiates the effects of another.

Physical interactions result when precipitation or another change in the physical state or solubility of a drug occurs. A common physical drug interaction takes place in the mixture of oppositely charged organic molecules [e.g., cationic (benzalkonium chloride) and anionic (soap) detergents].

Chemical drug interactions result when two administered substances combine with each other chemically. Tetracyclines complex with Ca (in milk), with aluminum (Al) and magnesium (Mg) (often components of antacids), and with Fe (in some multiple vitamins) to reduce the absorption of the tetracycline antibiotic.

25–27. The answers are 25-e, 26-b, 27-a. (*Hardman, pp 67–68. Katzung, pp 30, 134.*) Anaphylaxis refers to an acute hypersensitivity reaction that appears to be mediated primarily by immunoglobulin E (IgE). Specific antigens can interact with these antibodies and cause sensitized mast cells to release vasoactive substances, such as histamine. Anaphylaxis to penicillin is one of the best-known examples; the drug of choice to relieve the symptoms is epinephrine.

Decreased sensitivity to a drug, or tolerance, is seen with some drugs such as opiates and usually requires repeated administration of the drug. *Tachyphylaxis,* in contrast, is tolerance that develops rapidly, often after a single injection of a drug. In some cases, this may be due to what is termed as the *down regulation of a drug receptor,* in which the number of receptors becomes decreased.

A person who responds to an unusually low dose of a drug is called *hyperreactive.* Supersensitivity refers to increased responses to low doses only after denervation of an organ. At least three mechanisms are responsible for supersensitivity: (1) increased receptors, (2) reduction in tonic neuronal activity, and (3) decreased neurotransmitter uptake mechanisms.

28–30. The answers are 28-c, 29-a, 30-h. (*Katzung, pp 43–44.*) Time-action curves relate the changes in intensity of the action of a drug dose and the times that these changes occur. There are three distinct phases that characterize the time-action pattern of most drugs: (1) The time to onset of action is from the moment of administration (T on the figure that accompanies the question) to the time when the first drug effect is detected (U). (2) The time to reach the peak effect is from administration (T) until the maximum effect has occurred (W), whether this is above or below the level that produces some toxic effect. (3) The duration of action is described as the time from the appearance of a drug effect (U) until the effect disappears (Y). For some drugs, a fourth phase occurs (interval Y to Z), in which residual effects of the drug may be present. These are usually undetectable, but may be uncovered by readministration of the same drug dose (observed as an increase in potency) or by administration of another drug (leading to some drug-drug interaction).

31–33. The answers are 31-b, 32-a, 33-d. *(Katzung, pp 4–7.)* The absorption, distribution, and elimination of drugs require that they cross various cellular membranes. The descriptions that are given in the question define the various transport mechanisms. The most common method by which ionic compounds of low molecular weight (100 to 200) enter cells is via membrane channels. The degree to which such filtration occurs varies from cell type to cell type because their pore sizes differ.

Simple diffusion is another mechanism by which substances cross membranes without the active participation of components in the membranes. Generally, lipid-soluble substances employ this method to enter cells. Both simple diffusion and filtration are dominant factors in most drug absorption, distribution, and elimination.

Pinocytosis is a type of endocytosis that is responsible for the transport of large molecules such as proteins and colloids. Some cell types (e.g., endothelial cells) employ this transport mechanism extensively, but its importance in drug action is uncertain.

Membrane carriers are proteinaceous components of the cell membrane that are capable of combining with a drug at one surface of the membrane. The carrier-solute complex moves across the membrane, the solute is released, and the carrier then returns to the original surface where it can combine with another molecule of solute. There are two primary types of carrier-mediated transport: (1) active transport and (2) facilitated diffusion. During active transport, (1) the drug crosses the membrane against a concentration gradient, (2) the transport mechanism becomes saturated at high drug concentrations and thus shows a transport maximum, and (3) the process is selective for certain structural configurations of the drug. Active transport is responsible for the movement of a number of organic acids and bases across membranes of renal tubules, choroid plexuses, and hepatic cells. With facilitated diffusion, the transport process is selective and saturable, but the drug is not transferred against a concentration gradient and does not require the expenditure of cellular energy. Glucose transport into erythrocytes is a good example of this process. In both situations, if two compounds are transported by the same mechanism, one will competitively inhibit the transport of the other, and the transport process can be inhibited noncompetitively by substances that interfere with cellular metabolism.

34–36. The answers are 34-g, 35-a, 36-d. (*Katzung, pp 53–56.*) There are four major components to the mixed-function oxidase system: (1) cytochrome P450, (2) NADPH, or reduced nicotinamide adenine dinucleotide phosphate, (3) NADPH–cytochrome P450 reductase, and (4) molecular oxygen. The figure that follows shows the catalytic cycle for the reactions dependent upon cytochrome P450.

Cytochrome P450 catalyzes a diverse number of oxidative reactions involved in drug biotransformation; it undergoes reduction and oxidation during its catalytic cycle. A prosthetic group composed of Fe and protoporphyrin IX (forming heme) binds molecular oxygen and converts it to an activated form for interaction with the drug substrate. Similar to hemoglobin, cytochrome P450 is inhibited by carbon monoxide. This interaction results in an absorbance spectrum peak at 450 nm, hence the name P450.

NADPH gives up hydrogen atoms to the flavoprotein NADPH–cytochrome P450 reductase and becomes NADP+. The reduced flavoprotein transfers these reducing equivalents to cytochrome P450. The reducing

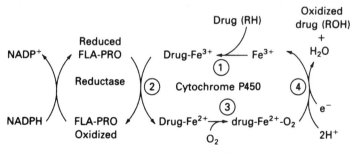

(From DiPalma and DiGregorio, with permission.)

equivalents are used to activate molecular oxygen for incorporation into the substrate, as described above. Thus, NADPH provides the reducing equivalents, while NADPH–cytochrome P450 reductase passes them on to the catalytic enzyme cytochrome P450.

MAO is a flavoprotein enzyme that is found on the outer membrane of mitochondria. It oxidatively deaminates short-chain monoamines only, and it is not part of the DMMS. ATP is involved in the transfer of reducing equivalents through the mitochondrial respiratory chain, not the microsomal system.

Anti-Infectives

Antibacterials
Antimycobacterials
Antifungals

Antivirals
Antiprotozoans

Questions

DIRECTIONS: Each item below contains a question or incomplete statement followed by suggested responses. Select the **one best** response to each question.

37. A 19-year-old male being treated for leukemia develops fever. You give agents that will cover bacterial, viral, and fungal infections. Two days later, he develops acute renal failure. Which drug was most likely responsible?

a. Vancomycin
b. Ceftazidime
c. Amphotericin B
d. Acyclovir

38. A 26-year-old female with acquired immunodeficiency syndrome (AIDS) develops cryptococcal meningitis. She refuses all intravenous medication. Which antifungal agent can be given orally to treat the meningeal infection?

a. Ketoconazole
b. Amphotericin B
c. Fluconazole
d. Nystatin

39. Why is vitamin B_6 usually prescribed with isoniazid (INH)?

a. It acts as a cofactor for INH
b. It prevents some adverse effects of INH therapy
c. Like INH, it has tuberculostatic activity
d. It prevents metabolism of INH

40. The quinolone derivative that is most effective against *Pseudomonas aeruginosa* is

a. Norfloxacin
b. Ciprofloxacin
c. Ofloxacin
d. Enoxacin
e. Lomefloxacin

41. A 19-year-old woman is diagnosed with tuberculosis (TB). Before prescribing a drug regimen, you take a careful medication history because one of the drugs commonly used to treat TB induces microsomal cytochrome P450 enzymes in the liver. Which drug is this?

a. Isoniazid
b. Rifampin
c. Pyrazinamide
d. Ethambutol
e. Vitamin B_6

42. The elimination half-life of which of the following tetracyclines remains unchanged when the drug is administered to an anuric patient?

a. Methacycline
b. Oxytetracycline
c. Doxycycline
d. Tetracycline
e. None of the above

43. In the treatment of bacterial meningitis in children, the drug of choice is

a. Penicillin G
b. Penicillin V
c. Erythromycin
d. Procaine penicillin
e. Ceftriaxone

44. In patients with hepatic coma, decreases in the production and absorption of ammonia from the gastrointestinal (GI) tract will be beneficial. The antibiotic of choice in this situation would be

a. Neomycin
b. Tetracycline
c. Penicillin G
d. Chloramphenicol
e. Cephalothin

45. Indicate from the diagram below the site of action of penicillinase.

a. A
b. B
c. C
d. D
e. E

46. Clavulanic acid is important because it

a. Easily penetrates Gram-negative microorganisms
b. Is specific for Gram-positive microorganisms
c. Is a potent inhibitor of cell-wall transpeptidase
d. Inactivates bacterial β-lactamases
e. Has a spectrum of activity similar to that of penicillin G

47. In the treatment of infections caused by *P. aeruginosa*, the antimicrobial agent that has proved to be effective is

a. Penicillin G
b. Piperacillin
c. Nafcillin
d. Erythromycin
e. Tetracycline

48. Ethambutol is administered concurrently with other antitubercular drugs in the treatment of TB in order to

a. Reduce the pain of injection
b. Facilitate penetration of the blood-brain barrier
c. Retard the development of organism resistance
d. Delay excretion of other antitubercular drugs by the kidney
e. Retard absorption after intramuscular injection

49. The most active aminoglycoside against *Mycobacterium tuberculosis* is

a. Streptomycin
b. Amikacin
c. Neomycin
d. Tobramycin
e. Kanamycin

50. The drug used in all types of TB is

a. Ethambutol
b. Cycloserine
c. Streptomycin
d. INH
e. PAS

51. Chronic candidiasis infections of the GI tract and oral cavity are treated with which agent in pill form

a. Amphotericin B
b. Nystatin
c. Miconazole
d. Fluconazole
e. Clotrimazole

52. Drug X is an antimycobacterial agent that inhibits other bacteria as well as poxviruses. However, it should not be used as a single agent because resistant mutants frequently form. The responsible mutation may alter the site of action of drug X [i.e., the deoxyribonucleic acid (DNA)–dependent ribonucleic acid (RNA) polymerase]. What is drug X?

a. INH
b. Rifampin
c. Pyrazinamide
d. Ethambutol

53. For the treatment of a patient with *Legionella pneumophila*, the drug of choice would be

a. Penicillin G
b. Chloramphenicol
c. Erythromycin
d. Streptomycin
e. Lincomycin

54. The most effective agent in the treatment of *Rickettsia, Mycoplasma,* and *Chlamydia* infections is

a. Penicillin G
b. Tetracycline
c. Vancomycin
d. Gentamicin
e. Bacitracin

55. The mechanism of action by which pyrantel pamoate is effective for the treatment of *Necator americanus* (hookworm) disease is

a. Interference with cell-wall synthesis
b. Interference with cell division
c. Inhibition of neuromuscular transmission
d. Interference with protein synthesis
e. Depletion of membrane lipoproteins

56. Vertigo, inability to perceive termination of movement, and difficulty in sitting or standing without visual clues are some of the toxic reactions that are likely to occur in about 75% of patients treated with

a. Penicillin G
b. Doxycycline
c. Amphotericin B
d. Streptomycin
e. INH

57. Amantadine, a synthetic antiviral agent used prophylactically against influenza A_2, is thought to act by

a. Preventing production of viral capsid protein
b. Preventing virion release
c. Preventing penetration of the virus into the host cell
d. Preventing uncoating of viral DNA
e. Causing lysis of infected host cells by release of intracellular lysosomal enzymes

58. Streptomycin and other aminoglycosides inhibit bacterial protein synthesis by binding

a. Peptidoglycan units in the cell wall
b. Messenger RNA (mRNA)
c. DNA
d. 30S ribosomal particles
e. RNA polymerase

59. A patient with AIDS is treated with a combination of agents, which includes zidovudine. What is the mechanism of action of zidovudine?

a. Inhibition of RNA synthesis
b. Inhibition of viral particle assembly
c. Inhibition of viral proteases
d. Inhibition of nucleoside reverse transcriptase
e. Inhibition of nonnucleoside reverse transcriptase

60. A 39-year-old male with aortic insufficiency and a history of no drug allergies is given an intravenous dose of antibiotic as a prophylaxis preceding the insertion of a valve prosthesis. As the antibiotic is being infused, the patient becomes flushed over most of his body. What antibiotic was given?
a. Vancomycin
b. Gentamicin
c. Erythromycin
d. Penicillin G
e. Tetracycline

61. Which of the following cephalosporins would have increased activity against anaerobic bacteria such as *Bacteroides fragilis?*
a. Cefaclor
b. Cephalothin
c. Cephalexin
d. Cefuroxime
e. Cefoxitin

62. Which one of the following antimicrobial agents is primarily administered topically?
a. Polymyxin B
b. Penicillin G
c. Dicloxacillin
d. Carbenicillin
e. Streptomycin

63. A 75-year-old woman is hospitalized for pneumonia and treated with an intravenous antibiotic. On day three, she develops severe diarrhea. Stool is positive for *Clostridium difficile* toxin. What is the best treatment?
a. Clindamycin
b. Cefaclor
c. Metronidazole
d. Erythromycin
e. Doxycycline

64. A jaundiced one-day-old premature infant with an elevated free bilirubin is seen in the premature-baby nursery. The mother received an antibiotic combination preparation containing sulfamethizole for a urinary tract infection (UTI) one week before delivery. You suspect that the infant's findings are caused by the sulfonamide because of the following mechanism:

a. Enhanced synthesis of bilirubin
b. Competition between the sulfonamide and bilirubin for binding sites on albumin
c. Inhibition of bilirubin degradation
d. Inhibition of urinary excretion of bilirubin

65. A 27-year-old female has just returned from a trip to Southeast Asia. In the past 24 hours, she has developed shaking, chills, and a temperature of 104°F. A blood smear reveals *Plasmodium vivax*. Which of the following agents should be used to eradicate the extraerythrocytic phase of the organism?

a. Primaquine
b. Pyrimethamine
c. Quinacrine
d. Chloroquine
e. Chloroguanide

66. An 86-year-old male complains of cough and blood in his sputum for the past two days. On admission, his temperature is 103°F. Physical examination reveals rales in his right lung, and x-ray examination shows increased density in the right middle lobe. A sputum smear shows many Gram-positive cocci, confirmed by sputum culture as penicillinase-producing *Staphylococcus aureus*. Which of the following agents should be given?

a. Ampicillin
b. Oxacillin
c. Carbenicillin
d. Ticarcillin
e. Mezlocillin

67. A 40-year-old male is HIV-positive with a cluster-of-differentiation-4 (CD4) count of 200/mm^3. Within two months, he develops a peripheral white blood cell count of 1000/mm^3 and a hemoglobin of 9.0 mg/dL. Which drug has most likely caused the adverse effect?

a. Acyclovir
b. Dideoxycytidine
c. Foscarnet
d. Rimantadine
e. Zidovudine

68. Thiabendazole, a benzimidazole derivative, is an antihelminthic drug used primarily to treat infections caused by

a. *Ascaris lumbricoides* (roundworm)
b. *N. americanus* (hookworm)
c. *Strongyloides*
d. *Enterobius vermicularis*
e. *Taenia saginata* (flatworm)

69. A 30-year-old male with a two-year history of chronic renal failure requiring dialysis consents to transplantation. A donor kidney becomes available. He is given cyclosporine to prevent transplant rejection just before surgery. What is the most likely adverse effect of this drug?

a. Bone marrow depression
b. Nephrotoxicity
c. Oral and GI ulceration
d. Pancreatitis
e. Seizures

70. The mechanism of action of chloroquine in *Plasmodium falciparum* malaria is elimination of

a. Secondary tissue schizonts
b. Exoerythrocytic schizonts
c. Erythrocytic stage
d. Asexual forms
e. Sporozoites

71. The use of chloramphenicol may result in

a. Bone marrow stimulation
b. Phototoxicity
c. Aplastic anemia
d. Staining of teeth
e. Alopecia

72. A drug primarily used in pneumonia caused by *Pneumocystis carinii* is

a. Nifurtimox
b. Penicillin G
c. Metronidazole
d. Pentamidine
e. Carbenicillin

DIRECTIONS: Each group of questions below consists of lettered options followed by a set of numbered items. For each numbered item, select the **one** lettered option with which it is **most** closely associated. Each lettered option may be used once, more than once, or not at all.

Questions 73–75

For each patient, select the mechanism of drug action:

a. Inhibition of bacterial cell-wall synthesis
b. Inhibition of bacterial protein synthesis
c. Inhibition of bacterial folic acid synthesis
d. Inhibition of bacterial topoisomerase II (DNA gyrase)
e. Inhibition of bacterial DNA polymerase

73. A 39-year-old female with a history of chronic UTI develops a new infection with *Escherichia coli* that is sensitive to levofloxacin.

74. A 25-year-old female with a sinus infection caused by *Haemophilus influenzae* is treated with trimethoprim-sulfamethoxazole.

75. A 35-year-old male has recently converted to positive on a purified protein derivative of tuberculin (PPD) test for TB. INH is given as prophylaxis.

76. Which of the following may cause damage to growing cartilage?

a. Fluoroquinolones
b. Sulfonamides
c. Aminoglycosides
d. Cephalosporins
e. Tetracyclines

77. A patient with AIDS is treated with a combination of agents, which includes efavirenz. What is the mechanism of action of efavirenz?

a. Inhibition of RNA synthesis
b. Inhibition of DNA synthesis
c. Inhibition of viral particle assembly
d. Inhibition of viral proteases
e. Inhibition of nucleoside reverse transcriptase
f. Inhibition of nonnucleoside reverse transcriptase

78. A patient with AIDS is treated with a combination of agents, which includes indinavir. What is the mechanism of action of indinavir?

a. Inhibition of RNA synthesis
b. Inhibition of DNA synthesis
c. Inhibition of viral particle assembly
d. Inhibition of viral proteases
e. Inhibition of nucleoside reverse transcriptase
f. Inhibition of nonnucleoside reverse transcriptase

79. Of the following, the most appropriate statement concerning the reactions caused by aminoglycosides is that these agents

a. Produce ototoxicity
b. Are potent neuromuscular blockers
c. Have little or no effect on kidneys
d. Produce a high incidence of hypersensitivity reactions similar to those of penicillins
e. Produce a high incidence of exfoliative dermatitis

Questions 80–81

For each patient, select the drug that most likely caused the adverse effect:

a. Acyclovir
b. Amantadine
c. Dideoxycytidine
d. Foscarnet
e. Ganciclovir
f. Idoxuridine
g. Interferon α
h. Ribavirin
i. Vidarabine
j. Zidovudine

80. A 27-year-old male with a three-year history of AIDS complains of progressive blurring of vision for two days. Eye examination reveals evidence of retinitis consistent with cytomegalic virus inclusion disease. Intravenous treatment is started, and within five days the patient complains of muscular weakness and cramping. Blood chemistries show a creatinine of 5.2 mEq/L and a Ca of 6.9 mEq/L.

81. A 22-year-old female with a two-year history of AIDS treated with one of these agents develops epigastric pain that radiates to the chest. Endoscopic examination reveals an esophageal ulceration.

82. The mechanism of action of chloramphenicol as an antibiotic is that it

a. Binds to the 30S ribosome subunit
b. Reversibly binds to the 50S ribosome subunit
c. Prevents cell membrane development
d. Inhibits cell-wall synthesis
e. Inhibits RNA polymerase

83. The drug of choice for the treatment of *T. saginata* (tapeworm) is

a. Mebendazole
b. Ceftriaxone
c. Primaquine
d. Niclosamide
e. Chloroquine

84. The drug of choice for the treatment of *Schistosoma haematobium* is

a. Praziquantel
b. Ceftriaxone
c. Metronidazole
d. Mebendazole
e. Diethylcarbamazine

85. Ampicillin and amoxicillin are in the same group of penicillins. Which of the following statements best characterizes amoxicillin?

a. It has better oral absorption than does ampicillin
b. It can be used in penicillinase-producing organisms
c. It is classified as a broad-spectrum penicillin
d. It does not cause hypersensitivity reactions
e. It is effective against *Pseudomonas*

86. A 60-year-old male with AIDS develops a systemic fungal infection that is treated with fluconazole. What is the mechanism of action of fluconazole?

a. It inhibits ergosterol synthesis
b. It inhibits DNA synthesis
c. It inhibits peptidoglycan synthesis
d. It inhibits protein synthesis

87. A 50-year-old male diabetic develops an external otitis from which *Pseudomonas* organisms are cultured. Topical therapy with polymyxin is effective. What is the mechanism of action of polymyxin?

a. Inhibition of cell-wall synthesis
b. Formation of reactive cytotoxic products that interfere with DNA synthesis
c. Disruption of membrane permeability
d. Inactivation of protein sulfhydryl groups
e. Inhibition of protein synthesis by binding to transfer RNA (tRNA)

88. A 75-year-old male develops a cough that produces blood-tinged sputum. He has a fever of 104°F. Gram-positive cocci in clusters are found in a sputum smear. A chest x-ray shows increased density in the right upper lobe. Of the following penicillins, which is most likely to be ineffective?

a. Oxacillin
b. Cloxacillin
c. Ticarcillin
d. Nafcillin
e. Dicloxacillin

89. A 40-year-old female with a history of AIDS develops a herpes simplex keratitis of the eye. Which of the following antiviral agents should be administered in this case?

a. Zanamivir
b. Trifluridine
c. Zidovudine
d. Amantadine
e. Indinavir

90. A 45-year-old female being treated for a chronic UTI develops acute alcohol intolerance. Which of the following agents could have caused this intolerance?

a. Cefoperazone
b. Amoxicillin
c. Sulfamethoxazole-trimethoprim
d. Norfloxacin
e. Tetracycline

91. A 60-year-old male with a temperature of 104°F and a productive cough is diagnosed as having staphylococcal pneumonia. After several days on nafcillin, he develops truncal urticaria and pruritis. Which of the following agents is best avoided in this patient?

a. Cefazolin
b. Clarithromycin
c. Sparfloxacin
d. Clindamycin
e. Tetracycline

92. A 65-year-old male with a pneumonia has a sputum culture that is positive for a staphylococcal strain that is β-lactamase-positive. Which is the best choice of penicillin therapy in this patient?

a. Ampicillin
b. Oxacillin
c. Ticarcillin
d. Penicillin G
e. Carbenicillin

93. A 35-year-old female complains of itching in the vulval area. Hanging-drop examination of the urine reveals trichomonads. What is the preferred treatment for trichomoniasis?

a. Doxycycline
b. Pyrimethamine
c. Pentamidine
d. Emetine
e. Metronidazole

94. A 40-year-old female with duodenal ulcers is treated with a combination of agents that includes clarithromycin. Of the following enzymes, which is inactivated by clarithromycin?

a. Dihydrofolate reductase
b. Glucose-6-phosphate dehydrogenase
c. Cytochrome P450
d. Na^+,K^+-ATPase
e. Na^+,K^+,Cl^- co-transporter

95. A 30-year-old type I diabetic with renal complications develops acute pyelonephritis. *P. aeruginosa* is found in urine cultures and blood cultures. Combined therapy is instituted with an aminoglycoside and which of the following?

a. Clavulanic acid
b. Vancomycin
c. A second-generation cephalosporin
d. Azithromycin
e. Piperacillin

96. A 35-year-old male is diagnosed with primary syphilis. Which of the following agents is the best choice for treating this patient?

a. A first-generation cephalosporin
b. Oxacillin
c. Imipenen
d. Benzathine penicillin G
e. Vancomycin

97. A 20-year-old male has a urethral discharge. Culture of the discharge shows *Neisseria gonorrhoeae.* Which of the following agents is the best choice for treating this patient?

a. Ceftriaxone
b. Benzathine penicillin G
c. Imipenen
d. Amikacin
e. Sulfamethoxazole-trimethoprim

98. Which of the following best describes ampicillin's effect on therapeutically administered estrogens?

a. It decreases estrogen metabolism
b. It decreases the enterohepatic circulation of estrogen
c. It decreases the plasma protein binding of estrogen
d. It decreases the renal excretion of estrogen
e. It decreases the sensitivity of estrogen at its site of action

99. A 36-year-old female with a chronic UTI treated with ciprofloxacin is not responsive to the antibiotic. Which of the following agents that she might have been taking for other reasons would decrease the effectiveness of ciprofloxacin?

a. An antacid
b. An antihistamine
c. A nonsteroidal anti-inflammatory
d. An anxiolytic
e. A multivitamin not containing iron

DIRECTIONS: Each group of questions below consists of lettered options followed by a set of numbered items. For each numbered item, select the **one** lettered option with which it is **most** closely associated. Each lettered option may be used once, more than once, or not at all.

Questions 100–101

For each of the parasites below, select the drug that is most effective against it.

a. Bithionol
b. Methotrexate
c. Pyrantel pamoate
d. Penicillin
e. Praziquantel
f. Ceftriaxone
g. Diethylcarbamazine
h. Primaquine
i. Niclosamide
j. Chloroquine

100. *A. lumbricoides* (roundworms)

101. *Wuchereria bancrofti* (filariae)

102. An infant with severe respiratory syncytial virus (RSV) bronchiolitis is best treated with

a. Amantadine
b. Indinavir
c. Efavirenz
d. Famciclovir
e. Ribavirin

103. A 20-year-old male with herpes simplex of the lips is treated with famciclovir. What is the mechanism of action of famciclovir?

a. Cross-linking of DNA
b. Strand breakage of DNA
c. Inhibition of viral DNA synthesis
d. Inhibition of nucleotide interconversions
e. Inhibition of a viral kinase

104. A 30-year-old pregnant female develops a UTI that is caused by *Chlamydia trachomatis*. Of the following, which is the best agent to use in this patient?

a. Tetracycline
b. Levofloxacin
c. Gentamycin
d. Erythromycin
e. Sulfamethoxazole-trimethoprim

105. A patient being treated with a combination of drugs for pulmonary tuberculosis develops a decrease in visual acuity and red-green color blindness resulting from retrobulbar neuritis. Which of the following agents is responsible for these findings?

a. INH
b. Streptomycin
c. Rifampin
d. Pyrizinamide
e. Ethambutol

Anti-Infectives

Answers

37. The answer is c. *(Hardman, p 1179. Katzung, pp 815–816.)* Amphotericin B may alter kidney function by decreasing creatinine clearance; if this occurs, the dose must be reduced. It also commonly increases potassium (K^+) clearance, leading to hypokalemia, and causes anemia and neurologic symptoms. A liposomal preparation may reduce the incidence of renal and neurologic toxicity. Vancomycin is less likely to cause kidney damage; if it does, the damage is less severe.

38. The answer is c. *(Hardman, p 1183. Katzung, p 819.)* Fluconazole penetrates into cerebrospinal fluid, where it is active against *Cryptococcus neoformans*. When it is given orally, blood levels are almost as high as when it is given parenterally. Amphotericin is administered intravenously and does not appear to be highly effective in fungal meningitis even when administered intrathecally.

39. The answer is b. *(Hardman, p 1158.)* Isoniazid inhibits cell-wall synthesis in mycobacteria. Increasing vitamin B_6 levels prevents complications associated with this inhibition, including peripheral neuritis, insomnia, restlessness, muscle twitching, urinary retention, convulsions, and psychosis, without affecting the antimycobacterial activity of INH.

40. The answer is b. *(Hardman, p 1065.)* Ciprofloxacin is a fluorinated quinolone derivative highly effective against *P. aeruginosa*. Other derivatives in this class have less activity toward this organism, although they are effective against other common Gram-negative organisms.

41. The answer is b. *(Katzung, pp 806–807.)* Rifampin induces cytochrome P450 enzymes, which causes a significant increase in elimination of drugs, such as oral contraceptives, anticoagulants, ketoconazole, cyclosporine, and chloramphenicol. It also promotes urinary excretion of methadone, which may precipitate withdrawal.

42. The answer is c. *(Hardman, pp 1129–1131.)* All tetracyclines can produce negative nitrogen balance and increased blood urea nitrogen

(BUN) levels. This is of clinical importance in patients with impaired renal function. With the exception of doxycycline, tetracyclines should not be used in patients that are anuric. Doxycycline is excreted by the GI tract under these conditions, and it will not accumulate in the serum of patients with renal insufficiency.

43. The answer is e. *(Hardman, pp 1094–1095.)* Penicillins were used in the treatment of meningitis because of their ability to pass across an inflamed blood-brain barrier. The third-generation cephalosporin, ceftriaxone, is preferred because it is effective against β-lactamase producing strains of *H. influenzae* that may cause meningitis in children.

44. The answer is a. *(Hardman, pp 1116–1117.)* Neomycin, an aminoglycoside, is not significantly absorbed from the GI tract. After oral administration, the intestinal flora is suppressed or modified and the drug is excreted in the feces. This effect of neomycin is used in hepatic coma to decrease the coliform flora, thus decreasing the production of ammonia that causes the levels of free nitrogen to decrease in the bloodstream. Other antimicrobial agents (e.g., tetracycline, penicillin G, chloramphenicol, and cephalothin) do not have the potency of neomycin in causing this effect.

45. The answer is e. *(Hardman, pp 1074–1076.)* Penicillinase hydrolyzes the β-lactam ring of penicillin G to form inactive penicilloic acid. Consequently, the antibiotic is ineffective in the therapy of infections caused by penicillinase-producing microorganisms such as staphylococci, bacilli, *E. coli, P. aeruginosa,* and *M. tuberculosis.*

46. The answer is d. *(Hardman, pp 1097–1098.)* The antibiotic clavulanic acid is a potent inhibitor of β-lactamases. The mode of inhibition is irreversible. Although clavulanic acid does not effectively inhibit the transpeptidase, it may be used in conjunction with a β-lactamase-sensitive penicillin to potentiate its activity.

47. The answer is b. *(Hardman, pp 1077–1086.)* Piperacillin is a broad-spectrum, semisynthetic penicillin for parenteral use. Its spectrum of activity includes various Gram-positive and Gram-negative organisms including *Pseudomonas.* The indications for piperacillin are similar to those for carbenicillin, ticarcillin, and mezlocillin, with the primary use being suspected or proven infections caused by *P. aeruginosa.* Penicillin G, nafcillin, erythromycin, and tetracycline are ineffective against *Pseudomonas.*

48. The answer is c. *(Hardman, pp 1161–1162.)* An important problem in the chemotherapy of TB is bacterial drug resistance. For this reason, concurrent administration of two or more drugs should be employed to delay the development of drug resistance. Isoniazid is often combined with ethambutol for this purpose. Streptomycin or rifampin may also be added to the regimen to delay even further the development of drug resistance.

49. The answer is a. *(Hardman, pp 1105–1108.)* The activity of streptomycin is bactericidal for the tubercle bacillus organism. Other aminoglycosides (e.g., gentamicin, tobramycin, neomycin, amikacin, and kanamycin) have activity against this organism but are seldom used clinically because of toxicity or development of resistance.

50. The answer is d. *(Hardman, pp 1155–1159.)* Only actively growing tubercle bacilli are susceptible to the bactericidal property of INH. The major action of INH is on the cell wall of the bacillus, where it prevents the synthesis of mycolic acid.

51. The answer is d. *(Hardman, pp 1183–1184.)* Mucocutaneous infections, most commonly *Candida albicans,* involve the moist skin and mucous membranes. Agents used topically include amphotericin B, nystatin, miconazole, and clotrimazole. Ketoconazole and fluconazole are administered orally in pill form for treatment of chronic infections.

52. The answer is b. *(Hardman, p 1159.)* Rifampin inhibits RNA synthesis in bacteria, mycobacteria, and chlamydiae by binding to the DNA-dependent RNA polymerase; it also inhibits assembly of poxvirus particles. Rifampin is used as a single prophylactic agent for contacts of people with meningococcal or *H. influenzae* type b infections. Otherwise, it is not used alone because 1 in 10 organisms in a population exposed to rifampin will become resistant, possibly because of mutation or a barrier against rifampin's entry into cells.

53. The answer is c. *(Hardman, pp 1135–1141.)* Erythromycin, a macrolide antibiotic, was initially designed to be used in penicillin-sensitive patients with streptococcal or pneumococcal infections. Erythromycin has become the drug of choice for the treatment of pneumonia caused by *Mycoplasma* and *Legionella*.

54. The answer is b. *(Hardman, p 1128.)* Tetracycline is one of the drugs of choice in the treatment of *Rickettsia, Mycoplasma,* and *Chlamydia* infections. The antibiotics that act by inhibiting cell-wall synthesis have no effect on *Mycoplasma* because the organism does not possess a cell wall; penicillin G, vancomycin, and bacitracin will be ineffective. Gentamicin has little or no antimicrobial activity with these organisms.

55. The answer is c. *(Hardman, p 1022.)* Pyrantel pamoate is an antihelminthic that acts primarily as a depolarizing neuromuscular blocker. In certain worms, a spastic neuromuscular paralysis occurs, resulting in the expulsion of the worms from the intestinal tract of the host. Pyrantel also exerts its effect against parasites via release of acetylcholine and inhibition of cholinesterase.

56. The answer is d. *(Hardman, pp 1110–1113.)* Streptomycin and other aminoglycosides can elicit toxic reactions involving both the vestibular and auditory branches of the eighth cranial nerve. Patients receiving an aminoglycoside should be monitored frequently for any hearing impairment owing to the irreversible deafness that may result from its prolonged use. None of the other agents listed in the question adversely affect the function of the eighth cranial nerve.

57. The answer is d. *(Katzung, p 840. Hardman, pp 1209–1211.)* Amantadine's mechanism of action involves inhibition of uncoating of the influenza A viral DNA. The primary target is the membrane M2 protein. The drug does not affect penetration and DNA-dependent RNA polymerase activity. Amantadine both reduces the frequency of illness and diminishes the serologic response to influenza infection. The drug has no action, however, on influenza B. As a weak base, amantadine buffers the pH of endosomes, thus blocking the fusion of the viral envelope with the membrane of the endosome.

58. The answer is d. *(Hardman, pp 1105–1108.)* The bactericidal activity of streptomycin and other aminoglycosides involves a direct action on the 30S ribosomal subunit, the site at which these agents both inhibit protein synthesis and diminish the accuracy of translation of the genetic code. Proteins containing improper sequences of amino acids (known as *nonsense proteins*) are often nonfunctional.

59. The answer is d. *(Katzung, pp 831–832.)* Zidovudine competitively inhibits HIV-1 nucleoside reverse transcriptase. It is also incorporated in the growing viral DNA chain to cause termination. Each action requires activation via phosphorylation of cellular enzymes. Zidovudine decreases the rate of clinical disease progression and prolongs survival in HIV-infected patients.

60. The answer is a. *(Hardman, p 1146.)* The "red man" syndrome is associated with vancomycin, thought to be caused by histamine release. Prevention consists of a slower infusion rate and pretreatment with antihistamines.

61. The answer is e. *(Hardman, pp 1092–1094.)* Cefoxitin and cefmetazole are suitable for treating intraabdominal infections. Such infections are caused by mixtures of aerobic and anaerobic Gram-negative bacteria like *B. fragilis.* Cefoxitin alone has been shown to be as effective as the traditional therapy of clindamycin plus gentamicin.

62. The answer is a. *(Hardman, pp 1143–1144.)* Polymyxin B is poorly absorbed by the oral route. It is primarily administered by the topical route for the treatment of infections of the skin, mucous membranes, eye, and ear. Penicillin G can be administered both orally and parenterally. Dicloxacillin is only given by the oral route. Carbenicillin and streptomycin are administered only by the parenteral route.

63. The answer is c. *(Hardman, pp 996–997, 1145–1146. Katzung, p 845.)* Metronidazole is often used to treat antibiotic-associated enterocolitis, especially when caused by *C. difficile.* Vancomycin is no longer preferred because it induces selection of resistant staphylococci. Clindamycin is also associated with *C. difficile* colitis, but in another way: a higher percentage of patients taking this over other antibiotics develop antibiotic-associated enterocolitis.

64. The answer is b. *(Hardman, p 1062.)* Sulfonamides should not be used in pregnant women who are at term because of their ability to cross the placenta and enter the fetus in concentrations sufficient to produce toxic effects. Sulfonamides should also not be given to neonates, especially premature infants, because they compete with bilirubin for serum albumin binding, resulting in increased levels of free bilirubin, which cause kernicterus.

65. The answer is a. *(Hardman, pp 977–978.)* Primaquine is effective against the extraerythrocytic forms of *P. vivax* and *P. ovale* and is thus of value in a radical cure of malarial infection. It also attacks the sexual forms of the parasite, rendering them incapable of maturation in the mosquito and making it valuable in preventing the spread of malarial infection.

66. The answer is b. *(Hardman, p 1077.)* Unlike the other listed drugs, oxacillin is resistant to penicillinase. The other four agents are broad-spectrum penicillins, while oxacillin is generally specific for Gram-positive microorganisms. Use of penicillinase-resistant penicillins should be reserved for infections caused by penicillinase-producing staphylococci.

67. The answer is e. *(Hardman, p 1206. Katzung, p 833.)* A major adverse effect of zidovudine is bone marrow depression that appears to be dose- and duration-dependent. The severity of the disease and a low CD4 count contribute to the bone marrow depression.

68. The answer is c. *(Hardman, p 1688.)* Thiabendazole has been shown to be effective against *Strongyloides,* cutaneous larva migrans, and *Trichuris.* Adverse effects consist of nausea, vertigo, headache, and weakness. Treatment usually involves oral administration for several days. It has been found to be ineffective in *Ascaris, N. americanus, E. vermicularis,* and *T. saginata.*

69. The answer is b. *(Hardman, p 1299. Katzung, p 609.)* Nephrotoxicity may occur in almost three-quarters of patients treated with cyclosporine. Regular monitoring of blood levels can reduce the incidence of adverse effects.

70. The answer is c. *(Hardman, pp 970–972.)* Chloroquine is a 4-aminoquinoline derivative that selectively concentrates in parasitized red blood cells. It is a weak base, and its alkalinizing effect on the acid vesicle of the parasite effectively destroys the viability of the parasite.

71. The answer is c. *(Hardman, pp 1134–1135.)* Hematologic toxicity is by far the most important adverse effect of chloramphenicol. The toxicity consists of two types: (1) bone marrow depression (common) and (2) aplastic anemia (rare). Chloramphenicol can produce a potentially fatal toxic reaction, the "gray baby" syndrome, caused by diminished ability of neonates to conjugate chloramphenicol with resultant high serum concentrations. Tetracyclines produce staining of the teeth and phototoxicity.

72. The answer is d. *(Hardman, p 989.)* Both trimethoprim-sulfamethoxazole and pentamidine are effective in pneumonia caused by *P. carinii.* This protozoal disease usually occurs in immunodeficient patients, such as those with AIDS. Nifurtimox is effective in trypanosomiasis and metronidazole in amebiasis and leishmaniasis, as well as in anaerobic bacterial infections. Penicillins are not considered drugs of choice for this particular disease state.

73. The answer is d. *(Hardman, pp 1065–1067. Katzung, p 797.)* Bacterial DNA gyrase is composed of four subunits, and levofloxacin binds to the strand-cutting subunits, inhibiting their activity.

74. The answer is c. *(Hardman, pp 1058–1059. Katzung, pp 793–795.)* Trimethoprim inhibits dihydrofolic acid reductase. Sulfamethoxazole inhibits *p*-aminobenzoic acid (PABA) from being incorporated into folic acid by competitive inhibition of dihydropteroate synthase. Either action inhibits the synthesis of tetrahydrofolic acid.

75. The answer is a. *(Hardman, p 1157. Katzung, p 804.)* Isoniazid inhibits mycobacterial cell-wall synthesis by inhibiting mycolic acid synthesis by a mechanism that is not fully understood.

76. The answer is a. *(Katzung, p 800.)* Fluoroquinolones are not recommended in patients less than 18 years old. They have a tendency to damage growing cartilage and cause arthropathy. The arthropathy is generally reversible. Tendinitis may occur, and in rare instances in adults, this finding may lead to tendon ruptures.

77. The answer is f. *(Katzung, p 837.)* Efavirenz is a specific inhibitor of HIV-1 viral growth. Its mechanism of action involves inhibition of nonnucleoside reverse transcriptase.

78. The answer is d. *(Katzung, p 839.)* Indinavir is a specific inhibitor of HIV-1 proteases. Cross-resistance can occur with other protease inhibitors.

79. The answer is a. *(Hardman, pp 1110–1111.)* All the aminoglycosides are potentially toxic to both branches of the eighth cranial nerve. The evidence indicates that the sensory receptor portions of the inner ear are affected rather than the nerve itself. Nephrotoxicity may develop during or after the use of an aminoglycoside. It is generally more common in the elderly when there is preexisting renal dysfunction. In most patients, renal function gradually improves after discontinuation of therapy. Aminoglycosides rarely cause neuromuscular blockade that can lead to progressive flaccid paralysis and potential fatal respiratory arrest. Hypersensitivity and dermatologic reactions occasionally occur following use of aminoglycosides.

80. The answer is d. *(Hardman, p 1200. Katzung, p 830.)* Nephrotoxicity and symptomatic hypocalcemia are major toxicities associated with foscarnet. Underlying renal disease, concomitant use of nephrotoxic drugs, dehydration, and rapid infusion of high doses increase the risk.

81. The answer is c. *(Katzung, p 835.)* Dideoxycytidine causes dose-dependent peripheral neuropathies and adverse effects in the GI tract, including nausea, diarrhea, and gastric and esophageal ulcerations and pancreatitis.

82. The answer is b. *(Hardman, p 1131.)* Chloramphenicol inhibits protein synthesis in bacteria and, to a lesser extent, in eukaryotic cells. The drug binds reversibly to the 50S ribosomal subunit and prevents attachment of aminoacyl-transfer RNA (tRNA) to its binding site. The amino acid substrate is unavailable for peptidyl transferase and peptide bond formation.

83. The answer is d. *(Hardman, p 1019.)* Niclosamide is a halogenated salicylanilide derivative. It exerts its effect against cestodes by inhibition of mitochondrial oxidative phosphorylation in the parasites. The mechanism of action is also related to its inhibition of glucose and oxygen uptake in the parasite.

84. The answer is a. *(Hardman, pp 1020–1022.)* Praziquantel is a broad-spectrum antihelminthic agent. It appears to kill the adult schistosome by increasing the permeability of the cell membranes of the parasite to Ca and consequent influx of Ca ions. This causes increased muscle contraction followed by paralysis.

85. The answer is a. *(Hardman, pp 1084–1085.)* Amoxicillin is classified as an aminopenicillin along with ampicillin. Because it is less affected than ampicillin by the presence of food, it has a superior absorption in the GI tract. It is sensitive to penicillinase and has a narrow spectrum of activity toward certain Gram-positive and Gram-negative organisms, but not *Pseudomonas.* Because it is in the penicillin family, hypersensitivity reactions are a possibility.

86. The answer is a. *(Hardman, p 1180. Katzung, pp 817–819.)* Fluconazole indirectly inhibits ergosterol synthesis. It inhibits cytochrome P450, which is a key enzyme system for cytochrome P450–dependent sterol 14-α-demethylase. This leads to accumulation of 14-α-sterols, resulting in impairment of the cytoplasmic membrane.

87. The answer is c. *(Hardman, pp 1143–1144.)* Bacitracin, cycloserine, cephalothin, and vancomycin inhibit cell-wall synthesis and produce bacteria that are susceptible to environmental conditions. Polymyxins disrupt the structural integrity of the cytoplasmic membranes by acting as cationic detergents. On contact with the drug, the permeability of the membrane changes. Polymyxin is often applied in a mixture with bacitracin and/or neomycin for synergistic effects.

88. The answer is c. *(Hardman, p 1086.)* Ticarcillin resembles carbenicillin and has a high degree of potency against *Pseudomonas* and *Proteus* organisms but is broken down by penicillinase produced by various bacteria, including most staphylococci. Oxacillin, cloxacillin, nafcillin, and dicloxacillin are all resistant to penicillinase and are effective against staphylococci.

89. The answer is b. *(Hardman, p 1203.)* Trifluridine inhibits viral activity in HSV types 1 and 2, CMV, vaccinia, and perhaps adenovirus. It acts as a viral DNA synthesis inhibitor by irreversibly blocking thymidylate synthetase. Trifluridine triphosphate is a competitive inhibitor of thymidine triphosphate accumulation into DNA. It is used in the treatment of primary keratoconjunctivitis and recurrent epithelial keratitis caused by HSV 1 and 2.

90. The answer is a. (*Hardman, pp 1086–1089.*) Intolerance of alcohol (disulfiram-like reaction) has been noted only with certain cephalosporins. Cephalosporins with the methylthiotetrazole side chain have been associated with a disulfiram-like reaction because the methylthiotetrazole group has a configuration similar to disulfiram, which blocks the metabolism of alcohol at the acetaldehyde step. Accumulation of acetaldehyde is associated with the symptoms. The methylthiotetrazole side chain also results in hypoprothrombinemia by interfering with the synthesis of vitamin K–dependent clotting factors.

91. The answer is a. (*Hardman, pp 1074–1077.*) Cephalosporins and penicillins have similar structures (they have a β-lactam ring), penicillins having a penicillic acid and the cephalosporins a cephalosporinic acid moiety. Both groups of antimicrobials inhibit the transpeptidase enzyme necessary for cross-linking of the peptidylglycan layer necessary for cell-wall stabilization. It appears that the mechanism is not totally identical for every drug for every bacterial species. Cephalosporins have a greater overall activity against Gram-negative organisms than do the penicillin G–type compounds. The hypersensitivity reactions associated with the penicillins and the cephalosporins appear to be identical in signs and symptoms. There is a crossover sensitivity between the penicillins and cephalosporins that must be considered when a patient is sensitive to either of these antibiotics. It occurs in about 5% to 10% of cases.

92. The answer is b. (*Hardman, p 1077.*) Oxacillin is classified as a penicillinase-resistant penicillin that is relatively acid-stable and, therefore, is useful for oral administration. Major adverse reactions include penicillin hypersensitivity and interstitial nephritis. With the exception of methicillin, which is 35% bound to serum proteins, all penicillinase-resistant penicillins are highly bound to plasma proteins. Oxacillin has a very narrow spectrum and is used primarily as an antistaphylococcal agent.

93. The answer is e. (*Hardman, pp 995–998.*) Metronidazole is a low-molecular-weight compound that penetrates all tissues and fluids of the body. Metronidazole's spectrum of activity is limited largely to anaerobic bacteria—including *B. fragilis*—and certain protozoa. It is considered to be the drug of choice for trichomoniasis in females and carrier states in males, as well as intestinal infections with *Giardia lamblia*.

94. The answer is c. *(Katzung, pp 778–780.)* Clarithromycin is a macrolide antibiotic. It can inhibit cytochrome P450. This could lead to an increase in concentration of drugs that are metabolized by cytochrome P450 and are given simultaneously with clarithromycin. When given with terfenadine, an antihistaminic agent, the interaction may lead to cardiac arrhythmias.

95. The answer is e. *(Katzung, p 761.)* Piperacillin is effective against *P. aeruginosa.* The ease with which these organisms develop resistance with single-drug therapy has necessitated that combination with aminoglycosides be used in pseudomonal infections.

96. The answer is d. *(Hardman, pp 1080–1082. Katzung, pp 759–760.)* Because of its long duration of action, benzathine penicillin G is given as a single injection of 1.2 million units intramuscularly every three or four weeks for the treatment of syphilis. This persistence of action reduces the need for repeated injections, costs, and local trauma. Benzathine penicillin G is also administered for group A, β-hemolytic streptococcal pharyngitis and pyoderma. For the later stages of syphilis, up to three weekly doses of the agent is administered.

97. The answer is a. *(Hardman, p 1082. Katzung, pp 764–766.)* The third-generation cephalosporin, ceftriaxone, and cefixime are considered first-line drugs in the treatment of gonorrhea because most strains of *Neisseria* gonococci are resistant to the penicillins. Amikacin and other aminoglycosides are used in serious infections caused by *E. coli, Enterobacter, Klebsiella,* and *Serratia* species. However, spectinomycin, which is related to the aminoglycosides, can be used as a backup drug for gonorrhea.

98. The answer is b. *(Katzung, p 1129.)* Ampicillin decreases the enterohepatic circulation of estrogen, thereby reducing its efficacy. It is thought that this occurs because of an alteration in the gastrointestinal flora. Other oral antibiotics may produce a similar effect.

99. The answer is a. *(Katzung, p 1124.)* Decreased gastrointestinal absorption of ciprofloxacin occurs with antacids because of their ability to adsorb the fluoroquinolone. Other preparations containing divalent ions, such as iron, will impede fluoroquinolone absorption.

100–101. The answers are 100-c, 101-g. (*Katzung, pp 879, 917–918.* *Hardman, pp 1010, 1022.*) Pyrantel is the drug of choice against *A. lumbricoides.* Its actions are as a depolarizing neuromuscular blocking agent and cholinesterase inhibitor. These actions cause spastic paralysis of the worms. Although benzimidazoles are also effective in treating *A. lumbricoides* and one of them could be considered the drug of choice, they have tetragenic potential. Filariasis is effectively treated with diethylcarbamazine, a piperazine derivative, which both suppresses and, in most cases, cures the infection. The drug is inactive against *W. bancrofti* in vitro. However, in vivo activity appears to be due to a sensitization of the microfilaria to phagocytosis by the fixed macrophages of the reticuloendothelial system.

102. The answer is e. (*Katzung, p 842.*) Ribavirin most likely interferes with guanosine triphosphate synthesis, resulting in inhibition of capping of viral messenger RNA and viral RNA-dependent RNA polymerase. It is effective in moderating infections with respiratory syncytial virus.

103. The answer is c. (*Katzung, pp 827–828.*) Famciclovir is active against herpes simplex and varicella zoster viruses. It is activated by a viral kinase to a triphosphate. The triphosphate is a competitive substrate for DNA polymerase. The incorporation of the famciclovir triphosphate into viral DNA results in chain termination.

104. The answer is d. (*Katzung, pp 779–780.*) Erythromycin is safe to use in pregnancy and is effective against *Chlamydia.* Levofloxacin is contraindicated in pregnancy because animal studies have identified that cartilage erosion can occur during growth. Chlamydia are not sensitive to gentamycin, however, it probably should not be used in pregnancy because of potential nephro- and ototoxicity. Tetracycline may cause tooth enamel dysplasia and problems with bone during fetal development. Sulfamethoxazole-trimethoprim has severe consequences, particularly in the newborn, because it displaces bilirubin from albumin, which is then deposited in the brain causing a condition referred to as *kernicterus.*

105. The answer is e. (*Katzung, p 807.*) Retrobulbar neuritis can occur with the use of ethambutol. It is dose related and typically occurs with prolonged therapy. The drug is not recommended for young children whose symptoms may not be easily assessed.

Cancer Chemotherapy and Immunology

Cell cycle
Alkylating agents
Hormones
Antibiotics
Antimetabolites

Plant alkaloids
Immunomodulators
Immunosuppressants
Radiopharmaceuticals

Questions

DIRECTIONS: Each item below contains a question or incomplete statement followed by suggested responses. Select the **one best** response to each question.

106. The most effective drug for immunosuppression of rejection of the allografted kidney is

a. Azathioprine
b. Cyclosporine
c. 5-fluorouracil (5-FU)
d. Cyclophosphamide
e. Vincristine

107. The phase of the cell cycle that is resistant to most chemotherapeutic agents and requires increased dosage to obtain a response is the

a. M phase
b. G_2 phase
c. S phase
d. G_0 phase
e. G_1 phase

108. A nucleophilic attack on deoxyribonucleic acid (DNA) that causes the disruption of base pairing occurs as a result of the administration of

a. Cyclophosphamide
b. 5-FU
c. Methotrexate
d. Prednisone
e. Thioguanine

109. The antineoplastic chemotherapeutic agent that is classified as an alkylating agent is

a. Thioguanine
b. Busulfan
c. Bleomycin
d. Vincristine
e. Tamoxifen

110. Which of the following is a chemotherapeutic drug that possesses a mechanism of action involving alkylation?

a. Cyclophosphamide
b. Methotrexate
c. Tamoxifen
d. 5-FU
e. Doxorubicin

111. A nine-year-old boy is diagnosed with acute lymphoblastic leukemia. He is maintained on methotrexate. A recent platelet count is below normal, and a stool guaiac is 4+. Which of the following agents should be administered to counteract methotrexate toxicity?

a. N-acetyl-L-cysteine
b. Vitamin K
c. Penicillamine
d. Leucovorin
e. Deferoxamine

112. Cardiotoxicity limits the clinical usefulness of which one of the following antitumor antibiotics?

a. Dactinomycin
b. Doxorubicin
c. Bleomycin
d. Plicamycin
e. Mitomycin

113. Binding to the enzyme dihydrofolate reductase is the mechanism of action for

a. Procarbazine
b. Paclitaxel
c. Methotrexate
d. Ifosfamide
e. Cladribine

114. Which of the following is considered to be the effective mechanism of action of the vinca alkaloids?

a. Inhibition of the function of microtubules
b. Damage and prevention of repair of DNA
c. Inhibition of DNA synthesis
d. Inhibition of protein synthesis
e. Inhibition of purine synthesis

115. The tumor that is least susceptible to cell-cycle-specific (CCS) anti-cancer agents is

a. Acute lymphoblastic leukemia
b. Acute granulocytic leukemia
c. Burkitt's lymphoma
d. Adenocarcinoma of the colon
e. Choriocarcinoma

116. A 32-year-old cancer patient, who has smoked two packs of cigarettes a day for 10 years, presents a decreased pulmonary function test. Physical examination and chest x-rays suggest preexisting pulmonary disease. Of the following drugs, which is best not prescribed?

a. Vinblastine
b. Doxorubicin
c. Mithramycin
d. Bleomycin
e. Cisplatin

117. Of the following, which is not a CCS agent

a. Mercaptopurine (6-MP)
b. 5-FU
c. Bleomycin
d. Busulfan
e. Vincristine

118. A 25-year-old female post–renal transplant shows signs of acute renal allograph rejection. Of the following agents, which should be administered?

a. Interferon α
b. Aldesleukin
c. Muromonab-CD3
d. Sargramostim
e. Filgrastim

119. A 50-year-old female with rheumatoid arthritis has developed erosions in her wrist bones. Which of the following agents should be administered?

a. Allopurinol
b. Asparaginase
c. Methotrexate
d. Streptozocin
e. 6-MP
f. Azathioprine
g. Pentostatin
h. Leucovorin
i. Bacille Calmette-Guérin (BCG) vaccine

120. A 40-year-old female post–renal transplant has developed evidence of osteoporosis, most likely due to cyclosporine. Which of the following agents might replace cyclosporine?

a. Allopurinol
b. Asparaginase
c. Methotrexate
d. Streptozocin
e. 6-MP
f. Azathioprine
g. Pentostatin
h. Leucovorin
i. BCG vaccine

121. A 34-year-old male with Hodgkin's disease is treated with the adriamycin, bleomycin, vinblastine, and decarbazine (ABVD) regimen. What is the mechanism of action of vinblastine?

a. Scission of DNA strands
b. Inhibition of dihydrofolate reductase
c. Inhibition of enzymes involved in purine metabolism
d. Prevention of assembly of tubulin dimers into microtubules
e. Inhibition of topoisomerase

122. A 60-year-old male with hematuria is found to have a small localized tumor of the bladder that is diagnosed as a carcinoma. Which of the following agents should be given intravesicularly?

a. Allopurinol
b. Asparaginase
c. Methotrexate
d. Streptozocin
e. 6-MP
f. Azathioprine
g. Pentostatin
h. Leucovorin
i. BCG vaccine

123. A 45-year-old female has a bone marrow transplant for treatment of ovarian cancer. Cyclosporine is given as an immunosuppressant. What is the mechanism of action of cyclosporine?

a. Direct destruction of proliferating lymphoid cells
b. Inhibition of T cell response to cytokines
c. Inhibition of folic acid metabolism
d. Inhibition of factors that stimulate T cell growth
e. Inhibition of enzymes that are related to purine metabolism

124. A young adult patient with acute granulocytic leukemia, treated with a combination of cytarabine and thioguanine, is no longer responsive to the therapy. The nonresponsiveness of the patient is thought to be due to thioguanine. What is the mechanism of resistance to thioguanine?

a. Decreased uptake
b. Increased efflux
c. Increased alkaline phosphatase activity
d. Increased production of trapping agents
e. Increased DNA repair

125. A 45-year-old male has an insulinoma. Which of the following agents is the treatment of choice?

a. Cyclophosphamide
b. Carboplatin
c. Vincristine
d. Streptozocin
e. Bleomycin

126. A 50-year-old female is treated with paclitaxel. Of the following, how is paclitaxel classified?

a. An alkylating agent
b. An antimetabolite
c. A plant alkaloid
d. An antibiotic
e. A hormonal agent

127. A 41-year-old female is treated for endometrial cancer with tamoxifen. Of the following, how is tamoxifen classified?

a. An alkylating agent
b. An antimetabolite
c. A plant alkaloid
d. An antibiotic
e. A hormonal agent

128. A 35-year-old female is being treated for cervical cancer with cisplatin. Of the following, how is cisplatin classified?

a. An alkylating agent
b. An antimetabolite
c. A plant alkaloid
d. An antibiotic
e. A hormonal agent

129. A 16-year-old male treated for acute lymphocytic leukemia develops severe lumbar and abdominal pain. His serum amylase is markedly elevated. Which of the following agents most likely caused these findings?

a. 6-MP
b. Asparaginase
c. Doxorubicin
d. Methotrexate
e. Vincristine

130. A 60-year-old female treated for breast cancer develops leukopenia and severe stomatitis and oral ulcerations. Which of the following agents most likely caused these findings?

a. 5-FU
b. Paclitaxel
c. Cyclophosphamide
d. Tamoxifen
e. Carboplatin

131. A 45-year-old male on combination therapy for remission-maintenance acute lymphocytic leukemia develops suprapubic pain, dysuria, and hematuria. Evidence of hemorrhage and inflammation is apparent on cystoscopy of the urinary bladder. Which of the following agents most likely caused these findings?

a. 6-MP
b. Methotrexate
c. Cyclophosphamide
d. Doxorubicin
e. Carmustine

132. A 45-year-old female treated for ovarian cancer develops difficulty hearing. Which of the following agents most likely caused these findings?

a. Paclitaxel
b. Doxorubicin
c. Bleomycin
d. 5-FU
e. Cisplatin

Questions 133–135

For each of the chemotherapeutic agents below, choose the phase of the cell cycle at which it is most likely to act.

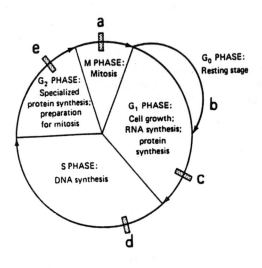

133. Busulfan

134. Methotrexate

135. Paclitaxel

Cancer Chemotherapy and Immunology

Answers

106. The answer is b. (*Hardman, pp 1296–1299.*) Cyclosporine is the preferred agent because it is a specific T cell inhibitor, and its success rate in protecting against rejection is considerably better than that of any other agent. All of the other agents listed in the question are cytotoxic. Because of the severe adverse reactions with cyclosporine, it is used in conjunction with azathioprine, which reduces the required dose. Prednisone is also used in conjunction with cyclosporine.

107. The answer is d. (*Katzung, pp 925–926. Hardman, pp 1231–1232.*) There are various phases described for the cell cycle. The M phase is the period of cell division (mitosis). Following the M phase, a cell may enter either the G_1 phase or G_0 phase. The G_1 phase of the cell cycle is associated with cell growth, ribonucleic acid (RNA) synthesis, and protein synthesis. The G_0 phase is the resting or dormant stage. No cell division takes place, although the cells are still capable of undergoing mitosis. This phase of the cell cycle is the most resistant to chemotherapeutic agents and may require a high dosage of the chemotherapeutic agent because most cancer drugs produce their lethal effect on cells that are actively involved in division. The S phase of the cell cycle involves DNA synthesis, and cells that are in the G_2 phase show the synthesis of specialized proteins in preparation for cell replication.

108. The answer is a. (*Hardman, p 1302.*) Cyclophosphamide, an alkylating agent, reacts with purine and pyrimidine bases of DNA to form bridges and dimers. These products interfere with DNA replication. 5-FU, methotrexate, and 6-thioguanine are antimetabolites, and the steroid prednisone has some tumor-suppressive effects.

109. The answer is b. (*Hardman, p 1241.*) Busulfan is an alkylating agent that, in contrast to other alkylators, is an alkylsulfonate. Thioguanine is a purine antimetabolite. Bleomycin is classified as a chemotherapeutic antibiotic, and vincristine is a vinca alkaloid. Tamoxifen is an antiestrogen hormone.

110. The answer is a. *(Hardman, p 1302.)* Cyclophosphamide is classified as a polyfunctional alkylating drug that transfers its alkyl groups to cellular components. The cytotoxic effect of this agent is directly associated with the alkylation of components of DNA. Methotrexate and 5-FU are classified as antimetabolites that block intermediary metabolism to inhibit cell proliferation. Tamoxifen is an antiestrogen compound. Doxorubicin is classified as an antibiotic chemotherapeutic agent.

111. The answer is d. *(Hardman, pp 1247, 1335.)* Leucovorin prevents methotrexate from inhibiting dihydrofolate reductase and reverses all of its adverse effects except neurotoxicity.

112. The answer is b. *(Hardman, pp 1264–1265.)* Dactinomycin's major toxicities include stomatitis, alopecia, and bone marrow depression. Bleomycin's toxicities include edema of the hands, alopecia, and stomatitis. Mitomycin causes marked bone marrow depression, renal toxicity, and interstitial pneumonitis. Plicamycin causes thrombocytopenia, leukopenia, liver toxicity, and hypocalcemia. The latter may be of use in the treatment of hypercalcemia. Doxorubicin causes cardiotoxicity, as well as alopecia and bone marrow depression. The cardiotoxicity has been linked to a lipid peroxidation within cardiac cells.

113. The answer is c. *(Hardman, pp 1243–1247.)* Antimetabolites of folic acid such as methotrexate, which is an important cancer chemotherapeutic agent, exert their effect by inhibiting the catalytic activity of the enzyme dihydrofolate reductase. The enzyme functions to keep folic acid in a reduced state. The first step in the reaction is the reduction of folic acid to 7,8-dihydrofolic acid (FH_2), which requires the cofactor nicotinamide adenine dinucleotide phosphate (NADPH). The second step is the conversion of FH_2 to 5,6,7,8-tetrahydrofolic acid (FH_4). This part of the reduction reaction requires nicotinamide adenine dinucleotide (NADH) or NADPH. The reduced forms of folic acid are involved in one-carbon transfer reactions that are required during the synthesis of purines and pyrimidine thymidylate. The affinity of methotrexate for dihydrofolate reductase is much greater than for the substrates of folic acid and FH_2. The action of methotrexate can be blocked or reduced by the administration of leuco-vorin (N^5-formyl FH$_4$), which can substitute for the reduced forms of folic acid in the cell. Methotrexate affects the S phase of the cell cycle. The drug is actively transported into the cell, and at very large doses the drug can enter the cell by simple diffusion. Although cladribine is an antimetabolite, it does not inhibit dihydrofolate reductase. Procarbazine, paclitaxel, and ifosfamide exert their anticancer effects through other mechanisms of action that are not associated with dihydrofolate reductase.

114. The answer is a. (*Hardman, pp 1259, 1260.*) The vinca alkaloids, vincristine and vinblastine, have proved valuable because they work on a different principle from most cancer chemotherapeutic agents. They (like colchicine) inhibit mitosis in metaphase by their ability to bind to tubulin. This prevents the formation of tubules and, consequently, the orderly arrangement of chromosomes, which apparently causes cell death.

115. The answer is d. (*Katzung, pp 925–926, 953.*) Cell-cycle-specific cytotoxic agents are most effective in malignancies in which a large portion of the population of malignant cells is undergoing mitosis. In leukemia, lymphoma, choriocarcinoma, and other rapidly growing tumors, these agents may induce a high-percentage cell kill of the entire tumor and at least of those cells that are actively dividing. In slowly growing, solid tumors, such as carcinomas of the colon, the frequency of actively dividing cells is low, and perhaps the resting cells survive the cycle-specific agents and then can be recruited back into the proliferative cycle.

116. The answer is d. (*Katzung, p 940. Hardman, p 1267.*) The potential serious adverse effect of bleomycin is pneumonitis and pulmonary fibrosis. This adverse effect appears to be both age- and dose-related. The clinical onset is characterized by decreasing pulmonary function, fine rales, cough, and diffuse basilar infiltrates. This complication develops in approximately 5% to 10% of patients treated with bleomycin. Thus, extreme caution must be used in patients with a preexisting history of pulmonary disease. All of the other drugs listed in the question are effective against carcinomas and have not been associated with significant lung toxicity.

117. The answer is d. (*Hardman, p 1236.*) Cell-cycle-specific agents such as 6-MP, 5-FU, bleomycin, and vincristine have proved to be the most effective against proliferating cells. Busulfan is an alkylating agent that binds to DNA and causes damage to these macromolecules. It is useful against low-growth, as well as high-growth, tumors and is classified as a cell-cycle-nonspecific (CCNS) agent.

118. The answer is c. *(Hardman, p 1302.)* Muromonab-CD3 is a monoclonal antibody that interferes with T cell function. It is classified as an immunosuppressive drug. This drug is given intravenously and is indicated in the treatment of acute allograft rejection. Generally, azathioprine and prednisone are used along with muromonab-CD3. Interferon α and aldesleukin (interleukin 2) are cytokines that are classified as immunostimulants. Sargramostim and filgrastim are also immunostimulants. These drugs are produced by recombinant DNA technology. Sargramostim is a human granulocyte-macrophage colony stimulating factor (GM-CSF), and filgrastim is a human granulocyte colony stimulating factor (G-CSF).

119. The answer is c. *(Katzung, pp 608–609, 932–933.)* Methotrexate is classified as an antimetabolite with therapeutic uses in cancer chemotherapy and as an immunosuppressive agent indicated in the treatment of severe active classical rheumatoid arthritis. Leucovorin is related to methotrexate in that it is an antagonist of its actions. It can supply a source of reduced folate for the methylation reactions that are prevented by methotrexate.

120. The answer is f. *(Katzung, p 972.)* Azathioprine is a derivative that is closely related to 6-MP, which is used as a cancer chemotherapeutic agent, while azathioprine is used as an immunosuppressive agent because it is more effective than 6-MP in this regard. Azathioprine is used in organ transplantation, particularly kidney allografts. Like 6-MP, azathioprine is biotransformed to an inactive product by xanthine oxidase. Allopurinol, which inhibits this enzyme, can increase the therapeutic action of azathioprine and possibly its adverse reactions. The dosage of azathioprine should be decreased in the presence of allopurinol.

121. The answer is d. *(Hardman, p 1258. Katzung, pp 935–936.)* Vinblastine binds to tubulin and blocks the protein from polymerizing to microtubules. The drug-tubulin complex binds to the developing microtubule, resulting in inhibition of microtubule assembly and subsequent depolymerization.

122. The answer is i. *(Katzung, p 984.)* Bacille Calmette-Guérin vaccine is a nonspecific stimulant of the reticuloendothelial system. It is an attenuated strain of *Mycobacterium bovis* that appears most effective in small, localized bladder tumors. This agent is approved for intravesicular use in bladder cancer. Adverse reactions are associated with the renal system, such as problems with urination, infection, and cystitis.

123. The answer is d. *(Katzung, p 969.)* Cyclosporine is a peptide antibiotic that both inhibits early stages of differentiation of T cells and blocks their activation. This most likely occurs in activated T lymphocytes by inhibition of gene transcription of immune-enhancing substances such as interferon γ and interleukins. Cyclophosphamide, an alkylating agent, destroys proliferating lymphoid cells. Sirolimus amarolide ab blocks the response of T cells to cytokines. Methotrexate is an inhibitor of folic acid synthesis. Azathioprine inhibits enzymes that are related to the biosynthesis of purines.

124. The answer is c. *(Katzung, p 933.)* Resistance to thioguanine occurs because of an increase in alkaline phosphatase and a decrease in hypoxanthine-guanine phosphoribosyl transferase. These enzymes are responsible, respectively, for the increase in dephosphorylation of thiopurine nucleotide and the conversion of thioguanine to its active form, 6-thioinosinic acid.

125. The answer is d. *(Hardman, pp 1242–1243.)* Streptozocin is an alkylating agent with the capacity to cross-link DNA, thereby inhibiting its synthesis. It is a nitrosourea-like antibiotic that contains a glucosamine moiety that allows it to be selectively taken up by the β cells of the islets of Langerhans. Consequently, it can be useful in treating metastatic islet cell carcinoma.

126. The answer is c. *(Hardman, pp 1260–1262.)* Paclitaxel is a large structural molecule that contains a 15-membered taxane ring system. This anticancer agent is an alkaloid derived from the bark of the Pacific yew tree. Its chemotherapeutic action is related to the microtubules in the cell. Paclitaxel promotes microtubule assembly from dimers and causes microtubule stabilization by preventing depolymerization. As a consequence of these actions, the microtubules form disorganized bundles, which decreases interphase and mitotic function. Furthermore, paclitaxel also causes premature cell division. The drug is administered intravenously and is useful in such diseases as cisplatin-resistant ovarian cancer, metastatic breast cancer, malignant melanoma, and acute myelogenous leukemia.

127. The answer is e. *(Katzung, pp 941–942.)* Tamoxifen is a partial antagonist of the estrogen receptor. It blocks the binding of estrogen to estrogen-sensitive cancer cells, particularly in breast cancer. It also acts effectively in progestin-resistant endometrial cancer.

128. The answer is a. *(Katzung, pp 931–932.)* Cisplatin is an inorganic metal complex that is thought to act in an analogous fashion as an alkylating agent. It inhibits DNA synthesis primarily through cross-linking of DNA and acts throughout the cell cycle. Binding of cisplatin occurs in DNA primarily with guanine residues, but interactions also can occur with adenosine and cytosine residues. It is used in bladder, testicular, and ovarian cancers.

129. The answer is b. *(Hardman, pp 1268–1269.)* Asparaginase is an enzyme that catalyzes the hydrolysis of serum asparagine to aspartic acid and ammonia. Major toxicities are related to antigenicity and pancreatitis. In addition, more than 50% of those treated present biochemical evidence of hepatic dysfunction.

130. The answer is a. *(Hardman, pp 1247–1251.)* 5-Fluorouracil is a pyrimidine antagonist that has a low neurotoxicity when compared with other fluorinated derivatives; however, its major toxicities are myelosuppression and oral or gastrointestinal ulceration. Leukopenia is the most frequent clinical manifestation of the myelosuppression.

131. The answer is c. *(Hardman, pp 1238–1239.)* Remission maintenance can be carried out by combination therapy, which includes cyclophosphamide. Cyclophosphamide causes hemorrhagic cystitis. Doxorubicin and carmustine are useful in the treatment of acute lymphatic leukemia, but neither is known to cause hemorrhagic cystitis.

132. The answer is e. *(Hardman, pp 1269–1271.)* Cisplatin causes acoustic nerve damage. Paclitaxel causes peripheral neuritis. Dose-dependent pneumonitis and fibrosis are caused by bleomycin. Doxorubicin causes cardiac toxicity, which may lead to congestive heart failure. 5-Fluorouracil causes myelosuppression, stomatitis, and oral and gastrointestinal ulcerations.

133–135. The answers are 133-b, 134-d, 135-a. *(Hardman, pp 1230–1232.)* Specific cell cycle events are present in both normal and cancerous cells. These phases of the cell cycle are shown in the diagram with the questions. Although general statements can be made regarding the cell cycle phases in which certain classes of chemotherapeutic agents act, some drugs listed in a particular category of antineoplastic agents may exhibit their effects on a different phase of the cell cycle. Alkylating agents are considered to be nonspecific in regard to the phase at which they have their effects. However, the alkylating agent busulfan is mostly active in the G_0 phase. S-phase-specific agents are cytosine arabinoside and hydroxyurea, while S-phase-specific agents that are self-limiting are 6-MP and methotrexate. M-phase-specific agents are vincristine, vinblastine, and paclitaxel. Antibiotic chemotherapeutic agents are considered to have effect in the G_2 phase of the cell cycle, with the exception of dactinomycin, which is most active in the S phase.

Cardiovascular and Pulmonary Systems

Agents for congestive heart failure
Antiarrhythmics
Antianginals
Antihypertensives
Anticoagulants
Antihyperlipidemics

Fibrinolytics
Procoagulants
Antianemics
Antiasthmatics
Mucokinetic agents

Questions

DIRECTIONS: Each question below contains several suggested responses. Select the **one best** response to each question.

136. The cardiovascular responses of a normal man were recorded and are shown in the accompanying figure following a 15-min infusion of drug X. Which of the following was most likely drug X?

a. Methacholine
b. Propranolol
c. Atropine
d. Isoproterenol
e. Norepinephrine

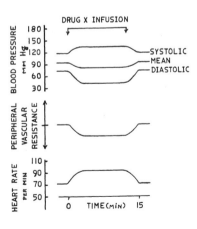

137. A 75-year-old female in congestive heart failure (CHF) is unable to climb a flight of stairs without experiencing shortness of breath. Digoxin is administered to improve cardiac muscle contractility. Within two weeks, she has a marked improvement in her symptoms. What cellular action of digoxin accounts for this?

   a. Inhibition of cyclic adenosine 5′-monophosphate (cAMP) synthesis
   b. Inhibition of mitochondrial calcium (Ca^{2+}) release
   c. Inhibition of the sodium (Na^+) pump
   d. Inhibition of β-adrenergic stimulation
   e. Inhibition of adenosine triphosphate (ATP) degradation

138. In a patient who has had attacks of paroxysmal atrial tachycardia, an ideal prophylactic drug is

   a. Adenosine
   b. Procainamide
   c. Lidocaine
   d. Nifedipine
   e. Verapamil

139. The therapeutic action of β-adrenergic receptor blockers such as propranolol in angina pectoris is believed to be primarily the result of

   a. Reduced production of catecholamines
   b. Dilation of the coronary vasculature
   c. Decreased requirement for myocardial oxygen
   d. Increased peripheral resistance
   e. Increased sensitivity to catecholamines

140. A 59-year-old female with mild CHF is treated with furosemide. What is its primary mechanism of action?

   a. Inhibition of sodium-potassium (Na^+,K^+) adenosine triphosphatase (ATPase)
   b. Inhibition of Na^+,K^+, chloride (Cl^-) co-transporter
   c. Inhibition of Na^+,Cl^- co-transporter
   d. Inhibition of Cl^- transporter
   e. Inhibition of Ca^{2+} divalent cation (Ca^{2+}) transporter

141. A positive Coombs' test and hemolytic anemia may follow the administration of which antihypertensive drug?

a. Methyldopa
b. Clonidine
c. Guanabenz
d. Prazosin
e. Captopril

142. Which of the following is an antiarrhythmic agent that has relatively few electrophysiologic effects on normal myocardial tissue but suppresses the arrhythmogenic tendencies of ischemic myocardial tissues?

a. Propranolol
b. Procainamide
c. Quinidine
d. Lidocaine
e. Disopyramide

143. A 59-year-old male with a history of rheumatic heart disease is found to have atrial fibrillation (AF), for which he is treated with digoxin. Treatment with digoxin converts his AF to a normal sinus rhythm and most likely results in a decrease in which of the following?

a. The length of the refractory period
b. The velocity of shortening of the cardiac muscle
c. The conduction velocity in the atrioventricular (AV) node
d. The atrial maximum diastolic resting potential

144. A 65-year-old female receives digoxin and furosemide for CHF. After several months, she develops nausea and vomiting. Serum K^+ is 2.5 mEq/L. Electrocardiogram (EKG) reveals an AV conduction defect. What cellular effect is causing these new findings?

a. Increased intracellular K^+
b. Increased intracellular cyclic guanosine 5'-monophosphate (cGMP)
c. Increased intracellular Ca^{2+}
d. Increased intracellular norepinephrine
e. Increased intracellular nitric oxide (NO)

145. Which of the following drugs recommended for the lowering of blood cholesterol inhibits the synthesis of cholesterol by blocking 3-hydroxy-3-methylglutaryl–coenzyme A (HMG-CoA) reductase?

   a. Lovastatin
   b. Probucol
   c. Clofibrate
   d. Gemfibrozil
   e. Nicotinic acid (NA)

146. The EKG of a patient who is receiving digitalis in the therapeutic dose range would be likely to show

   a. Prolongation of the QT interval
   b. Prolongation of the PR interval
   c. Symmetric peaking of the T wave
   d. Widening of the QRS complex
   e. Elevation of the ST segment

147. A 45-year-old male takes simvastatin for hypercholesterolemia; however, his cholesterol level remains above target at maximal doses. Cholestyramine is added to the therapeutic regimen. What drug-drug interaction can occur?

   a. The combination will not lower cholesterol more than either agent alone
   b. The combination causes elevated very-low-density lipoprotein (VLDL)
   c. Cholestyramine inhibits gastrointestinal (GI) absorption of simvastatin
   d. Simvastatin is a direct antagonist of cholestyramine

148. In a hypertensive patient who is taking insulin to treat diabetes, which of the following drugs is to be used with extra caution and advice to the patient?

   a. Hydralazine
   b. Prazosin
   c. Guanethidine
   d. Propranolol
   e. Methyldopa

149. Which of the following drugs is considered to be most effective in relieving and preventing ischemic episodes in patients with variant angina?

a. Propranolol
b. Nitroglycerin
c. Sodium nitroprusside
d. Nifedipine
e. Isosorbide dinitrate

150. A 47-year-old male is seen in the medicine clinic with recently diagnosed mixed hyperlipidemia. An antihyperlipidemic is administered that favorably affects levels of VLDL, low-density lipoprotein (LDL), and high-density lipoprotein (HDL) and inhibits cholesterol synthesis. This drug is:

a. Lovastatin
b. Colestipol
c. Niacin
d. Probucol
e. Neomycin

151. If quinidine and digoxin are administered concurrently, which of the following effects does quinidine have on digoxin?

a. The absorption of digoxin from the GI tract is decreased
b. The metabolism of digoxin is prevented
c. The concentration of digoxin in the plasma is increased
d. The effect of digoxin on the AV node is antagonized
e. The ability of digoxin to inhibit the Na^+ K^+-stimulated ATPase is reduced

152. Drugs that block the catecholamine uptake process (e.g., cocaine, tricyclic antidepressants, and phenothiazines) are apt to block the antihypertensive action of which of the following drugs?

a. Propranolol
b. Guanethidine
c. Prazosin
d. Hydralazine
e. Diazoxide

153. A 44-year-old obese male has a significantly high level of plasma triglycerides. Following treatment with one of the following agents, his plasma triglyceride levels decrease to almost normal. Which agent did he receive?

a. Neomycin
b. Lovastatin
c. Cholestyramine
d. Gemfibrozil

154. A 64-year-old male with arteriosclerotic heart disease (AHD) and CHF who has been treated with digoxin complains of nausea, vomiting, and diarrhea. His EKG reveals a bigeminal rhythm. The symptoms and EKG findings occurred shortly after another therapeutic agent was added to his regimen. A drug-drug interaction is suspected. Which agent was involved?

a. Lovastatin
b. Hydrochlorothiazide
c. Phenobarbital
d. Nitroglycerin
e. Captopril

155. Nicotinic acid in large doses used to treat hyperlipoproteinemia causes a cutaneous flush. The vasodilatory effect is due to

a. Release of histamine
b. Production of local prostaglandins
c. Release of platelet-derived growth factor (PDGF)
d. Production of NO
e. Ca channel blockade

156. One type of hyperlipoproteinemia is characterized by elevated plasma levels of chylomicra, normal plasma levels of β-lipoproteins, and the inability of any known drug to reduce lipoprotein levels. This is which of the following types of hyperlipoproteinemia?

a. Type I
b. Type IIa, IIb
c. Type III
d. Type IV
e. Type V

157. A 69-year-old male with angina develops severe constipation following treatment with

a. Propranolol
b. Captopril
c. Verapamil
d. Dobutamine
e. Nitroglycerin

158. Angiotensin converting enzyme (ACE) inhibitors are associated with a high incidence of which of the following adverse reactions?

a. Hepatitis
b. Hypokalemia
c. Agranulocytosis
d. Proteinuria
e. Hirsutism

159. A 45-year-old male post–myocardial infarction (post-MI) for one week is being treated with intravenous (IV) heparin. Stool guaiac on admission was negative, but is now 4+, and he has had an episode of hematemesis. The heparin is discontinued, and a drug is given to counteract the bleeding. What drug was given?

a. Aminocaproic acid
b. Dipyridamole
c. Factor IX
d. Protamine
e. Vitamin K

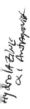

160. Patients with genetically low levels of N-acetyltransferase are more prone to develop a lupus erythematosus–like syndrome with which of the following drugs?

a. Propranolol
b. Procainamide
c. Digoxin
d. Captopril
e. Lidocaine

161. Which of the following anemias would be treated with cyanocobalamin (vitamin B$_{12}$)?

a. Anemia in infants who are undergoing rapid growth
b. Anemia associated with cheilosis, dysphagia, gastritis, and hypochlorhydria
c. Anemia associated with small, bizarre cells poorly filled with hemoglobin
d. Anemia associated with infestation by *Diphyllobothrium latum*
e. Bleeding from a gastric ulcer

162. The preferred agent to combat extreme digoxin overdose is

a. K$^+$
b. Ca^{2+}
c. Phenytoin
d. Fab fragments of digoxin antibodies
e. Magnesium (Mg^{2+})

163. Significant relaxation of smooth muscle of both venules and arterioles is produced by which of the following drugs?

a. Hydralazine
b. Minoxidil
c. Diazoxide
d. Sodium nitroprusside
e. Nifedipine

164. Precautions advisable when using lovastatin include

a. Serum transaminase measurements
b. Renal function studies
c. Acoustic measurements
d. Monthly complete blood counts
e. Avoidance of bile acid sequestrants

165. The first-line drug for treating an acute attack of reentrant supraventricular tachycardia (SVT) is

a. Adenosine
b. Digoxin
c. Propranolol
d. Phenylephrine
e. Edrophonium

Questions 166–168

For each patient, select the drug most likely to have caused the changes.

a. Acetazolamide
b. Amiloride
c. Furosemide
d. Hydrochlorothiazide
e. Mannitol

166. An 83-year-old male has been effectively treated with hydrochloro-thiazide to control his elevated blood pressure. He has had a recent onset of weakness. Blood chemistry analysis reveals a K^+ of 2.5 mEq/L. Another drug is added, and one month later his serum K^+ is 4.0 mEq/L. *b*

b

167. A 76-year-old male with a combined history of bronchiogenic carci-noma and CHF is maintained on a diuretic to control pulmonary and peripheral edema. Recent measurement of blood electrolytes reveals an ele-vated serum Ca^{2+}. *d*

168. A 66-year-old female with CHF and hearing loss is given a diuretic as part of a regimen that includes digoxin and an ACE inhibitor. In the course of treatment, she develops an AV conduction defect and is found to be hypomagnesemic. She also has worsening hearing loss, which is reversed when the drug is stopped. *c*

169. A 60-year-old male, following hospitalization for an acute myocar-dial infarction, is treated with warfarin. What is the mechanism of action of warfarin? *c*

a. Increase in the plasma level of factor IX
b. Inhibition of thrombin and early coagulation steps
c. Inhibition of synthesis of prothrombin and coagulation factors VII, IX, and X
d. Inhibition of platelet aggregation in vitro
e. Activation of plasminogen
f. Binding of Ca^{2+} ion cofactor in some coagulation steps

170. A 39-year-old pregnant female requires heparin for thromboembolic phenomena. What is the mechanism of action of heparin?

  a. Increase in the plasma level of factor IX
  b. Inhibition of thrombin and early coagulation steps
  c. Inhibition of synthesis of prothrombin and coagulation factors VII, IX, X
  d. Inhibition of platelet aggregation in vitro
  e. Activation of plasminogen
  f. Binding of Ca^{2+} ion cofactor in some coagulation steps

171. A 42-year-old male with an acute MI is treated with alteplase. What is the mechanism of action of alteplase?

  a. Inhibition of platelet thromboxane production
  b. Antagonism of ADP receptor
  c. Glycoprotein IIb/IIIa antagonist
  d. Inhibition of the synthesis of vitamin K–dependent coagulation factors
  e. Activation of plasminogen from plasmin

172. A 65-year-old male with a previous history of a stroke is treated with ticlopidine as prophylaxis for preventing further stroke. What is the mechanism of action of ticlopidine?

  a. Inhibition of platelet thromboxane production
  b. Antagonism of ADP receptor
  c. Antagonism of glycoprotein IIb/IIIa
  d. Inhibition of the synthesis of vitamin K–dependent coagulation factors
  e. Activation of plasminogen to plasmin

173. A 40-year-old female is to have angioplasty following an acute MI. As part of her treatment, she is given intravenously administered eptifibatide. What is the mechanism of action of eptifibatide?

  a. Inhibition of platelet thromboxane production
  b. Antagonism of ADP receptor
  c. Antagonism of glycoprotein IIb/IIIa
  d. Inhibition of the synthesis of vitamin K–dependent coagulation factors
  e. Activation of plasminogen from plasmin

174. Administration of which of the following antianginal agents results in antianginal effects for only 10 hours, despite detectable therapeutic plasma levels for 24 hours?

 a. Atenolol
 b. Transdermal nitroglycerin
 c. Amlodipine
 d. Amyl nitrite

175. A 70-year-old female is treated with sublingual nitroglycerin for her occasional bouts of angina. Which of the following is involved in the action of nitroglycerin?

 a. α-adrenergic activity
 b. Phosphodiesterase activity
 c. Phosphorylation of light chains of myosin
 d. Norepinephrine release
 e. cGMP

176. A 56-year-old female has recently developed essential hypertension, for which she is receiving chlorothiazide to lower her blood pressure. Which of these ions would not increase in concentration in her urine?

 a. K^+
 b. Cl^-
 c. Ca^{2+}
 d. Na^+
 e. Mg^{2+}

177. A 60-year-old female with deep-vein thrombosis (DVT) is given a bolus of heparin, and a heparin drip is also started. Thirty minutes later, she is bleeding profusely from the intravenous site. The heparin is stopped, but the bleeding continues. You decide to give protamine to reverse the adverse effect of heparin. How does protamine act?

 a. It causes hydrolysis of heparin
 b. It changes the conformation of antithrombin III to prevent binding to heparin
 c. It activates the coagulation cascade, overriding the action of heparin
 d. It combines with heparin as an ion pair, thus inactivating it

178. A 47-year-old female comes to the emergency department (ED) with severe crushing chest pain of one hour's duration. Electrocardiogram and blood chemistries are consistent with a diagnosis of acute MI. Streptokinase is chosen as part of the therapeutic regimen. What is its mechanism of action?

    a. It activates the conversion of fibrin to fibrin-split products
    b. It activates the conversion of plasminogen to plasmin
    c. It inhibits the conversion of prothrombin to thrombin
    d. It inhibits the conversion of fibrinogen to fibrin

Questions 179–181

For each patient, select the drug most likely to have caused the adverse effect.

    a. Adenosine
    b. Captopril
    c. Clonidine
    d. Digoxin
    e. Dobutamine
    f. Furosemide
    g. Guanethidine
    h. Lidocaine
    i. Nifedipine
    j. Prazocin
    k. Procainamide
    l. Propranolol

179. A 36-year-old male is seen in the ED with tachycardia, a respiratory rate of 26 breaths per minute (BPM), and EKG evidence of an arrhythmia. An intravenous bolus dose of an antiarrhythmic agent is administered, and within 30 s, he has a respiratory rate of 45 BPM and complains of a burning sensation in his chest.

180. Following a cardiac triple-bypass operation, a 65-year-old normotensive hospitalized female has shortness of breath, diffuse rales bilaterally, a pulse of 110/min, an elevated venous pressure, and a blood pressure of 140/85 mmHg. An intravenous dose of drug is given to counteract her findings. However, following administration of this drug, her pulse increases to 150/min and her blood pressure to 180/110 mmHg.

181. A 50-year-old male with a two-year history of essential hypertension well controlled on hydrochlorothiazide is found on a recent physical examination to have a blood pressure of 160/105 mmHg. The hydrochlorothiazide is substituted with another agent. Two weeks later, he returns for follow-up complaining of a loss of taste.

182. A 54-year-old female is treated for essential hypertension with an antihypertensive that controls her blood pressure. One day, she comes to the ED with chest pain, tachycardia, anxiety, and a blood pressure of 240/140 mmHg. She has not taken her medication for two days. Which antihypertensive can account for her findings?

a. Clonidine
b. Propranolol
c. Doxazosin
d. Minoxidil
e. Prazosin

Questions 183–184

For each patient, select the drug most likely to have caused the adverse effect.

a. Adenosine
b. Amiodarone
c. Bretylium
d. Flecainide
e. Procainamide
f. Propafenone
g. Quinidine
h. Sotalol
i. Tocainide
j. Verapamil

183. A 68-year-old female has AF, which is treated with an antiarrhythmic agent that blocks Na^+ channels. On a recent office visit, she complained of recurrent attacks of feeling faint and of experiencing an episode of loss of consciousness. An EKG showed marked prolongation of the QT interval. Plasma concentration of the drug was in the therapeutic range.

184. A 55-year-old male has recurrent ventricular arrhythmias after an MI, for which he is given an antiarrhythmic agent that blocks Na^+ channels and prolongs the action potential. One year later, a blood test is positive for circulating antinuclear antibodies.

Questions 185–187

Match each treatment indication with the correct drug.

a. Isoproterenol
b. Sotalol
c. Nitroglycerin
d. Amiodarone
e. Beclomethasone
f. Sodium nitroprusside

185. Angina pectoris

186. Myocardial stimulation

187. Bronchial asthma

Questions 188–189

It is customary today to classify antiarrhythmic drugs according to their mechanism of action. This is best defined by intracellular recordings that yield monophasic action potentials. In the accompanying figure, the monophasic action potentials of (A) slow response fiber (SA node) and (B) fast Purkinje fiber are shown. For each description that follows, choose the appropriate drug with which the change in character of the monophasic action potential is likely to be associated.

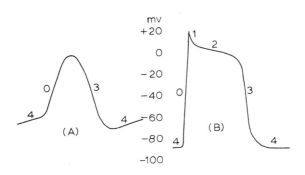

a. Digoxin
b. Amiodarone
c. Mexiletine
d. Nifedipine
e. Propranolol
f. Flecainide
g. Disopyramide *Nor paro*
h. Verapamil

188. Moderate phase 0 depression and slow conduction; prolonged repolarization   *g*

189. Affects mainly phase 3, prolonging repolarization   *b*

190. A 60-year-old male with chronic obstructive lung disease is given ipratropium as part of his therapeutic regimen. What is the mechanism of action of ipratropium?

a. Inhibition of airway muscarinic receptors
b. Inhibition of 5-lipoxygenase
c. Breakdown of mucus
d. Inhibition of mediator release
e. Inhibition of phosphodiesterase
f. Activation of β-adrenergic receptors

191. A one-year-old male develops decreased breath sounds, and wheezing during a febrile episode, which is relieved by albuterol. What is the mechanism of action of albuterol?

a. Inhibition of airway muscarinic receptors
b. Inhibition of 5-lipoxygenase
c. Breakdown of mucus
d. Inhibition of mediator release
e. Inhibition of phosphodiesterase
f. Activation of β-adrenergic receptors

192. A 10-year-old female with allergy-induced asthma is treated with cromolyn. What is the mechanism of action of cromolyn?

a. Inhibition of airway muscarinic receptors
b. Inhibition of 5-lipoxygenase
c. Breakdown of mucus
d. Inhibition of mediator release
e. Inhibition of phosphodiesterase
f. Activation of β-adrenergic receptors

193. Which of the following is unlikely to occur with low concentrations of nitroglycerin?

a. Decreased heart rate
b. Decreased end-diastolic blood pressure
c. Decreased myocardial oxygen demand
d. Decreased preload and afterload
e. Increased coronary blood flow

194. A 40-year-old male with markedly elevated cholesterol, diagnosed as having heterozygous familial hypercholesterolemia, is treated with cholestyramine. What is the mechanism of action of cholestyramine?

- a. Sequestration of bile acids
- b. Decreased hepatic secretion of VLDL
- c. Increased lipoprotein lipase activity
- d. Inhibition of HMG-CoA reductase
- e. Decreased oxidation of plasma lipids

195. A 35-year-old male with markedly elevated plasma triglyceride and LDL levels, and low plasma HDL levels, is treated with gemfibrozil. What is the mechanism of action of gemfibrozil?

- a. Sequestration of bile acids
- b. Decreased hepatic secretion of VLDL
- c. Increased lipoprotein lipase activity
- d. Inhibition of HMG-CoA reductase
- e. Decreased oxidation of plasma lipids

Questions 196–197

Match the descriptions below with the appropriate agent.

- a. Angiotensin I
- b. Angiotensin II
- c. Clonidine
- d. Losartan
- e. Captopril

196. Formed by sequential enzymatic cleavage by renin and then peptidyl dipeptidase (kinase II)   *B*

197. Lowers blood pressure in hypertensive patients by inhibition of peptidyl dipeptidase   *e*

198. A 65-year-old male post-MI with an elevated LDL level is treated with atorvastatin. What is the mechanism of action of atorvastatin?

- a. Sequestration of bile acids
- b. Decreased hepatic secretion of VLDL
- c. Increased lipoprotein lipase activity
- d. Inhibition of HMG-CoA reductase
- e. Decreased oxidation of plasma lipids

199. A 76-year-old female with an eight-year history of CHF that has been well controlled with digoxin and furosemide develops recurrence of dyspnea on exertion. On physical examination, she has sinus tachycardia, rales at the base of both lungs, and 4+ pitting edema of the lower extremities. Which agent could be added to her therapeutic regimen?

a. Dobutamine
b. Hydralazine
c. Minoxidil
d. Prazosin
e. Enalapril

200. A 61-year-old female has intermittent bouts of chest pain on exertion of two months' duration, associated with numbness and tingling in the fourth and fifth fingers of her left hand. An EKG is normal. She is placed on propranolol, which relieves her symptoms. What cardiovascular effect did the drug have?

a. It decreased production of catecholamines
b. It dilated the coronary vasculature
c. It decreased the requirement for myocardial oxygen
d. It increased peripheral vascular resistance
e. It increased sensitivity to catecholamines

201. The blood pressure of a 65-year-old male is well controlled by a Ca^{2+} channel blocker that is used to treat his essential hypertension. When placed on cimetidine to control symptoms related to gastroesophageal reflux disease (GERD), he has episodes of dizziness. How does cimetidine's effect on Ca^{2+} channel blockers account for the dizziness?

a. It increases their rate of intestinal absorption
b. It decreases their plasma protein binding
c. It decreases their volume of distribution
d. It decreases their metabolism by cytochrome P450
e. It decreases their tubular renal secretion

202. Which of the following best describes cimetidine's mechanism of interaction with procainamide?
   a. It decreases procainamide metabolism
   b. It decreases procainamide sensitivity at the site of action
   c. It decreases procainamide renal excretion
   d. It decreases procainamide plasma protein binding
   e. It decreases procainamide intestinal absorption

203. Which of the following best describes diltiazem's effect on digoxin?
   a. It decreases digoxin metabolism
   b. It decreases digoxin renal excretion
   c. It decreases digoxin plasma protein binding
   d. It decreases digoxin intestinal absorption
   e. It decreases digoxin sensitivity at its site of action

204. Which of the following best describes the mechanism of kaolin-pectin's interaction with digoxin?
   a. It decreases digoxin metabolism
   b. It decreases digoxin renal excretion
   c. It decreases digoxin plasma protein binding
   d. It decreases digoxin intestinal absorption
   e. It decreases digoxin sensitivity at its site of action

Cardiovascular and Pulmonary Systems

Answers

136. The answer is d. *(Hardman, pp 212–213.)* Only isoproterenol will lower mean blood pressure, decrease peripheral vascular resistance, and increase heart rate. Methacholine decreases heart rate as does propranolol. Atropine has no action on peripheral resistance. Norepinephrine causes intense vasoconstriction and raises the mean blood pressure.

137. The answer is c. *(Hardman, p 810.)* Digitalis inhibits Na^+,K^+-ATPase and, hence, decreases myocyte Na pumping, resulting in a relative reduction of Ca expulsion from Na-Ca exchange. The consequent increase in free Ca in the cell causes an increased intensity of interaction between actin and myosin filaments and enhanced contractility.

138. The answer is e. *(Hardman, pp 858–874.)* Because verapamil, a Ca channel blocker, has a selective depressing action on AV nodal tissue, it is an ideal drug for both immediate and prophylactic therapy of supraventricular tachycardia (SVT). Nifedipine, another Ca channel blocker, has little effect on SVT. Lidocaine and adenosine are parenteral drugs with short half-lives and, thus, are not suitable for prophylactic therapy. Procainamide is more suitable for ventricular arrhythmias and has the potential for serious adverse reactions with long-term use.

139. The answer is c. *(Hardman, pp 855–856.)* β-adrenergic receptor blockers cause a slowing of heart rate, lower blood pressure, and lessened cardiac contractility without reducing cardiac output. There is also a buffering action against adrenergic stimulation of the cardiac autoregulatory mechanism. These hemodynamic actions decrease the requirement of the heart for oxygen.

140. The answer is b. *(Hardman, p 697.)* The primary action of furosemide is inhibition of the Na^+,K^+,Cl^- transporter in the thick ascending limb of the loop of Henle.

141. The answer is a. (*Katzung, p 162.*) Many drugs can cause an immunohemolytic anemia. Methyldopa may cause a positive Coombs' test in as many as 20% of patients, along with hemolytic anemia. Other drugs with similar actions on red blood cells are penicillins, quinidine, procainamide, and sulfonamides. These form a stable or unstable hapten on the red cell surface, which induces an immune reaction [immunoglobulin G (IgG) antibodies] and leads to dissolution of the membrane.

142. The answer is d. (*Hardman, pp 865–867.*) Lidocaine usually shortens the duration of the action potential and, thus, allows more time for recovery during diastole. It also blocks both activated and inactivated Na channels. This has the effect of minimizing the action of lidocaine on normal myocardial tissues as contrasted with depolarized ischemic tissues. Thus, lidocaine is particularly suitable for arrhythmias arising during ischemic episodes such as myocardial infarction (MI).

143. The answer is c. (*Hardman, pp 813–814.*) Digoxin is used in AF to slow the ventricular rate, not usually the AF itself. Digoxin acts to slow the speed of conduction, increase the atrial and AV nodal maximal diastolic resting membrane potential, and increase the effective refractory period in the AV node, which prevents transmission of all impulses from the atria to the ventricles. It exerts these effects by acting directly on the heart and by indirectly increasing vagal activity.

144. The answer is c. (*Katzung, pp 225–227.*) Overloading of cell Ca leads to *delayed afterdepolarizations*. These afterpotentials can interfere with normal conduction by further reducing the resting potential; if they regularly reach threshold in the conduction system, an arrhythmia can occur.

145. The answer is a. (*Hardman, pp 885–887.*) Lovastatin decreases cholesterol synthesis in the liver by inhibiting HMG-CoA reductase, the rate-limiting enzyme in the synthetic pathway. This results in an increase in LDL receptors in the liver, thus reducing blood levels for cholesterol. The intake of dietary cholesterol must not be increased, as this would allow the liver to use more exogenous cholesterol and defeat the action of lovastatin.

146. The answer is b. (*Hardman, pp 813–814.*) The usual electrocardiographic pattern of a patient receiving therapeutic doses of digitalis includes an increase in the PR interval, depression and sagging of the ST segment, and occasional biphasia or inversion of the T wave. Symmetrically peaked T waves are associated with hyperkalemia or ischemia in most cases. Shortening of the QT interval, rather than prolongation, is characteristic of digitalis treatment.

147. The answer is c. *(Hardman, pp 887, 889.)* Bile acid-binding resins bind more than just bile acids, and binding of simvastatin to cholestyramine is the most likely mechanism for decreased GI absorption. Cholestyramine may also bind to several other drugs, including digoxin, benzothiadiazines (thiazides), warfarin, vancomycin, thyroxine (T_4), and aspirin. Medications should be given one hour before or four hours after cholestyramine.

148. The answer is d. *(Hardman, pp 855–856.)* Propranolol, as well as other nonselective beta blockers, tends to slow the rate of recovery in a hypoglycemic attack caused by insulin. Beta blockers also mask the symptoms of hypoglycemia and may actually cause hypertension because of the increased plasma epinephrine in the presence of a vascular $beta_2$ blockade.

149. The answer is d. *(Hardman, pp 767–775.)* Ca channel blockers, of which nifedipine is a prime example, are now considered to be more effective than nitrates in relieving variant angina. This is because this type of angina is believed to be caused by vasospasm, which is best antagonized by slow-channel Ca blockers. Such blockers appear to have a relative selectivity for coronary arteries.

150. The answer is c. *(Hardman, p 890. Katzung, pp 588–589.)* Only niacin improves levels of VLDL, HDL, and LDL and inhibits cholesterol synthesis. It also limits the progression of atherosclerosis by lowering circulating fibrinogen and increasing circulating tissue plasminogen activator (tPA).

151. The answer is c. *(Hardman, pp 870–871.)* Quinidine is often given in conjunction with digitalis. It has been found by pharmacokinetic studies that this combination results in quinidine's replacing digitalis in tissue binding sites (mainly muscle), thus raising the blood level of digitalis and decreasing its volume of distribution. A mechanism by which quinidine interferes with the renal excretion of digitalis has also been proposed.

152. The answer is b. *(Hardman, p 790.)* Neuronal uptake is necessary for the hypotensive action of guanethidine. It competes for the norepinephrine storage site and, in time, replaces the natural neurotransmitter. This is the basis of its hypotensive effect. Drugs that prevent reuptake by the neurons, such as cocaine, would destroy the effectiveness of guanethidine.

153. The answer is d. *(Katzung, pp 589–590.)* Only gemfibrozil acts to lower triglycerides, probably because of increased lipolysis by lipoprotein lipase and decreased lipolysis inside adipocytes, causing a net movement of triglycerides into the cell.

154. The answer is b. *(Hardman, pp 703–704.)* Low K stores due to the effects of thiazide diuretics such as hydrochlorothiazide increase susceptibility to cardiac glycoside toxicity.

155. The answer is b. *(Hardman, pp 890–891.)* Nicotinic acid in large doses stimulates the production of prostaglandins as shown by an increase in blood level. The flush may be prevented by the prior administration of aspirin, which is known to block synthesis of prostaglandins.

156. The answer is a. *(Hardman, pp 875–898.)* In type I hyperlipoproteinemia, drugs that reduce levels of lipoproteins are not useful, but reduction of dietary sources of fat may help. Cholesterol levels are usually normal, but triglycerides are elevated. Maintenance of ideal body weight is recommended in all types of hyperlipidemia. Clofibrate effectively reduces the levels of VLDLs that are characteristic of types III, IV, and V hyperlipoproteinemia; administration of cholestyramine resin and lovastatin in conjunction with a low-cholesterol diet is regarded as effective therapy for type IIa, or primary, hyperbetalipoproteinemia, except in the homozygous familial form.

157. The answer is c. *(Katzung, p 239. Hardman, pp 772–773.)* Constipation, particularly severe with verapamil, may occur with Ca channel blockers. In addition, excessive vasodilation may also occur. This can cause dizziness, hypotension, headache, flushing, nausea, and diminished sensation in fingers and toes. Constipation, lethargy, nervousness, and peripheral edema are also seen with the use of Ca channel blockers.

158. The answer is d. *(Hardman, p 750.)* The most consistent of the toxicities of ACE inhibitors is impairment of renal function, as evidenced by proteinuria. Elevations of blood urea nitrogen (BUN) and creatinine occur frequently, especially when stenosis of the renal artery or severe heart failure exists. Hyperkalemia also may occur. These drugs are to be used very cautiously where prior renal failure is present and in the elderly. Other toxicities include persistent dry cough, neutropenia, and angioedema. Hepatic toxicity has not been reported.

159. The answer is d. *(Hardman, p 1346.)* A slow intravenous infusion of protamine sulfate will quickly reverse the bleeding. Protamine binds to heparin to form a stable complex with no anticoagulant activity. It may also have its own anticoagulant effect by binding with platelets and fibrinogen.

160. The answer is b. *(Hardman, pp 868–869.)* Persons with low hepatic N-acetyltransferase activity are known as *slow acetylators*. A major pathway of metabolism of procainamide, which is used to treat arrhythmias, is N-acetylation. Slow acetylators receiving this drug are more susceptible than normal persons to side effects, because slow acetylators will have higher-than-normal blood levels of these drugs. N-acetylprocainamide, the metabolite of procainamide, is also active.

161. The answer is d. *(Hardman, pp 1331–1333.)* Iron-deficiency anemia usually occurs in infants undergoing rapid growth. In adults in a late stage, it may result in a bowel syndrome associated with gastritis and hypochlorhydria (Plummer-Vinson syndrome). Characteristically, all iron-deficiency anemias are associated with a hypochromic microcytic blood profile. Infestation with the tapeworm *D. latum* is accompanied by a hyperchromic macrocytic anemia, which is treatable with vitamin B_{12}. Bleeding syndromes are treated with iron.

162. The answer is d. *(Hardman, p 820.)* In digoxin overdose, only the administration of a specific Fab fragment that acts as an antibody for digoxin is effective. This raises the blood level of the digoxin, but it is not available for action on the heart and, indeed, the combined Fab fragment–digoxin complex is excreted by the kidney. While K, Mg, and phenytoin will counteract some of the arrhythmogenic actions of digoxin, they are not effective in severe digoxin overdose. Calcium would augment the toxicity of digoxin.

163. The answer is d. *(Hardman, pp 794–795.)* Hydralazine, minoxidil, diazoxide, and sodium nitroprusside are all directly acting vasodilators used to treat hypertension. Because hydralazine, minoxidil, nifedipine, and diazoxide relax arteriolar smooth muscle more than smooth muscle in venules, the effect on venous capacitance is negligible. Sodium nitroprusside, which affects both arterioles and venules, does not increase cardiac output, a feature that enhances the utility of sodium nitroprusside in the management of hypertensive crisis associated with MI.

164. The answer is a. *(Hardman, pp 885–887.)* Lovastatin should not be used in patients with severe liver disease. With routine use of lovastatin, serum transaminase values may rise, and in such patients the drug may be continued only with great caution. Lovastatin has also been associated with lenticular opacities, and slit-lamp studies should be done before and one year after the start of therapy. There is no effect on the otic nerve. The drug is not toxic to the renal system, and reports of bone marrow depression are very rare. There is a small incidence of myopathy, and levels of creatinine kinase should be measured when unexplained muscle pain occurs. Combination with cyclosporine or clofibrate has led to myopathy. There is no danger in use with bile acid sequestrants.

165. The answer is a. *(Katzung, p 240.)* Older therapies—all designed to favor parasympathetic control of rhythm—include digoxin, propranolol, edrophonium, and vasoconstrictors. The vasoconstrictor phenylephrine (given by intravenous bolus) causes stimulation of the carotid sinus and reflex vagal stimulation of the atria. More recently, adenosine has been favored over verapamil, which is also very effective but slower acting.

166. The answer is b. *(Katzung, pp 256–258.)* Amiloride is a K-sparing diuretic with a mild diuretic and natriuretic effect. The parent compound is active, and the drug is excreted unchanged in the urine. Amiloride has a 24-hour duration of action and is usually administered with a thiazide or loop diuretic (e.g., furosemide) to prevent hypokalemia. The site of its diuretic action is the late distal tubule and collecting duct, where it interferes with Na reabsorption and allows for K retention.

167. The answer is d. *(Katzung, pp 254–256.)* Thiazide diuretics raise serum Ca, possibly through a direct effect on Ca reabsorption in the distal tubule. While rarely caused by the diuretic alone, hypercalcemia can occur when the patient has a history of carcinoma.

168. The answer is c. *(Katzung, pp 252–254.)* Furosemide can cause hypokalemia by blocking Na^+ reabsorption in the loop of Henle, followed by exchange of K^+ with Na^+ in the distal tubules. Hypokalemia is associated with digitalis toxicity. Furosemide also can cause dose-related hearing loss, especially in people with existing hearing loss and/or renal impairment.

169. The answer is c. *(Hardman, pp 1347–1348. Katzung, p 570.)* Warfarin is a coumarin derivative that is generally used for chronic anticoagulation. It antagonizes the γ carboxylation of several glutamate residues in prothrombin and the coagulation factors VII, IX, and X. This process is coupled to the oxidative deactivation of vitamin K. The reduced form of vitamin K is essential for sustained carboxylation and synthesis of the coagulation proteins. It appears that warfarin inhibits the action of the reductase(s) that regenerate the reduced form of vitamin K. The prevention of the inactive vitamin K epoxide from being reduced to the active form of vitamin K results in decreased carboxylation of the proteins involved in the coagulation cascade.

170. The answer is b. *(Hardman, p 1344. Katzung, pp 567–568.)* Heparin binds to antithrombin III (a plasma protease inhibitor), thereby enhancing its activation. The heparin–antithrombin III complex interacts with thrombin. This inactivates thrombin and other coagulation factors such as VIIa, IXa, Xa, and IIa. Heparin accelerates the rate of thrombin-antithrombin binding, resulting in the inhibition of thrombin. The latter effect is not typically seen with low-molecular-weight heparins that are not of sufficient length to catalyze the inhibition of thrombin.

171. The answer is e. *(Katzung, pp 572–574.)* Alteplase is an unmodified tPA. Alteplase activates plasminogen that is bound to fibrin. The plasmin that is formed acts directly on fibrin. This results in dissolving the fibrin into fibrin-split products followed by lysis of the clot.

172. The answer is b. *(Katzung, pp 574–575.)* Ticlopidine inhibits platelet aggregation and the release of platelet granule constituents. It does this by inhibiting the binding of ADP to its platelet receptor. Platelet membrane function is altered irreversibly by inhibition of ADP-induced activation of the platelet glycoprotein GPIIb/IIIa complex, resulting in decreased fibrinogen binding. Decreased platelet aggregation stems from the inability of activated platelets to recruit circulating platelets. Clopidogrel is relatively newer than ticlopidine. It appears to be as effective as ticlopidine and has fewer side effects.

173. The answer is c. *(Katzung, p 575.)* Eptifibatide is a cyclic heptapeptide that binds to platelet glycoprotein IIb/IIIa. This prevents the binding of fibrinogen to the platelet glycoprotein IIb/IIIa receptor. Its peak action occurs within an hour and is maintained during the infusion period. The effect is reversible within four to eight hours following infusion.

174. The answer is b. *(Katzung, p 189.)* Significant tolerance to nitroglycerin develops. Transdermal patches can produce therapeutic drug levels for 24 hours, but its effectiveness lasts between 8 and 10 hours. A nitrate-free period of at least eight hours is necessary to prevent tolerance. Amyl nitrite is inhalable, and its action lasts no longer than five minutes. Patients on atenolol and amlodipine do not develop tolerance to these agents.

175. The answer is e. *(Katzung, p 184. Hardman, p 764.)* Nitric oxide is thought to be enzymatically released from nitroglycerin. It can then react with and activate guanylyl cyclase to increase GMP, a vasodilator due to its effect on increasing calcium efflux. It also indirectly causes the dephosphorylation of the light chains of myosin. These actions lead to the vasodilator effect of nitroglycerin. Reaction of nitric oxide occurs with protein sulfhydryl groups. Tolerance may develop in part from a decrease in available sulfhydryl groups. Autonomic receptors are not involved in the primary response of nitroglycerin, but compensatory mechanisms may counter the primary actions.

176. The answer is c. (*Katzung, pp 254–255.*) Thiazide diuretics enhance K, Cl, Na, and Mg ion excretion; Ca excretion appears to be reduced following chronic drug administration. Because thiazides inhibit NaCl reabsorption in the early portion of the distal tubule, an increased load of Na and Cl ions is presented to the collecting duct, where some Na ions may be actively reabsorbed and K ions secreted, leading to increased K loss.

177. The answer is d. (*Hardman, p 1346.*) Heparin is a mixture of sulfated mucopolysaccharides and is highly acidic and highly charged. Protamine is a very basic polypeptide that combines with heparin. The complex has no anticoagulant activity. Excess protamine does have anticoagulant activity, so just enough should be given to counteract the heparin effect.

178. The answer is b. (*Hardman, p 1352.*) Streptokinase forms a stable complex with plasminogen. The resulting conformational change allows for formation of free plasmin, the active fibrinolytic enzyme.

179. The answer is a. (*Hardman, p 858. Katzung, p 240.*) Many patients that receive a therapeutic dose of adenosine experience shortness of breath and fullness or a burning sensation in the chest. These adverse effects are of short duration because of rapid elimination of the drug.

180. The answer is e. (*Hardman, p 213.*) Intravenous infusion of dobutamine may result in an increased heart rate and blood pressure. Patients with a history of hypertension are more likely to have an exaggerated blood pressure response.

181. The answer is b. (*Hardman, pp 750–751.*) Angiotensin converting enzyme inhibitors, especially captopril, can cause alteration or loss of taste sensation.

182. The answer is a. (*Hardman, p 789. Katzung, pp 162–163.*) Withdrawal of clonidine, particularly doses greater than 1 mg/d, is well known to cause such a syndrome (including severe hypertension, tachycardia, anxiety, tremor, headache, abdominal pain, and sweating), even after one or two missed doses.

183. The answer is g. *(Hardman, p 870. Katzung, pp 230–231.)* Quinidine causes prolongation of the QT interval at therapeutic doses, possibly because of its antimuscarinic actions. In some patients, this is associated with recurrent lightheadedness and fainting (known as *quinidine syncope*). The symptoms result from torsades de pointes. They typically terminate but may become fatal by degeneration into ventricular fibrillation.

184. The answer is e. *(Hardman, p 868. Katzung, pp 231–232.)* Procainamide blocks open Na^+ channels. Long-term therapy can result in drug-induced lupus syndrome, identified by circulating antinuclear antibodies. Many patients may develop a facial rash and joint pains. Pericarditis can occur, but renal involvement is rare.

185–187. The answers are 185-c, 186-a, 187-e. *(Hardman, pp 212, 214, 666, 764, 800.)* The coronary vasodilator nitroglycerine may be administered orally, sublingually, topically, intravenously, and most recently transdermally. Its small dose and molecular structure permit its passage through the skin. This is accomplished by attaching a nitroglycerine-containing, multilayered film to the skin. Isoproterenol, a catecholamine that acts on β-adrenergic receptors, is given parenterally because absorption after sublingual or oral administration is unreliable. It is a synthetic sympathomimetic, structurally similar to epinephrine. Isoproterenol produces myocardial stimulation and is used for the treatment of AV heart block, cardiogenic shock associated with MI, cardiac arrest, and septicemic shock. Beclomethasone is a glucocorticoid especially designed for aerosol administration. This permits its therapeutic action in the lungs while minimizing systemic effects. Great care must be exercised when transferring patients from systemic corticosteroids to beclomethasone because fatal adrenal insufficiency has occurred in asthmatic patients undergoing such transfer.

188–189. The answers are 188-g, 189-b. *(Hardman, pp 858–859, 864–865.)* It is widely accepted that antiarrhythmic drugs are best classified according to their electrophysiologic attributes. This is best accomplished by relating the effects of the different drugs to their actions on Na and Ca channels, which are reflected by changes in the monophasic action potential. Amiodarone blocks Na, Ca, and K currents and markedly prolongs repolarization, particularly in depolarized cells. Flecainide is related to local anesthetics and also affects Na channels, but has little effect on repolarization. Mexiletine, which is in the same group of local anesthetics as lidocaine, is remarkable because it either does not affect or shortens repolarization. Its action is mainly on depolarized fibers. Disopyramide slows depolarization and repolarization and, like quinidine, delays conduction. Verapamil, a Ca channel blocker, affects the resting potential, or phase 4, and thus has its greatest effect on pacemaker tissue; it is mainly of utility in supraventricular arrhythmias. Digitalis also affects phase 4 of the action potential, but it also greatly hastens repolarization. Although nifedipine is a Ca channel blocker, it has little effect on the electrophysiology of the heart. Propranolol has actions mainly on slow-response fibers and suppresses automaticity.

190. The answer is a. (*Katzung, pp 342–343.*) Ipratropium is a muscarinic receptor antagonist. It is a quaternary ammonium derivative of atropine. It is not readily absorbed, allowing for the delivery of relatively high concentrations to muscarinic receptors in the airways. Compared with atropine, adverse effects are minimal, particularly because there is almost no absorption into the central nervous system (CNS). Muscarinic receptor antagonists are used to replace β-adrenergic agonists in those patients that show intolerance to them and prove to be effective in chronic obstructive lung disease.

191. The answer is f. (*Katzung, pp 340–341.*) Albuterol is a short-acting β-adrenergic agonist. It is effective in obtaining immediate relief and is delivered by inhalation in acute episodes of bronchospasm. Its action may last up to four hours. Salmeterol is a long-acting β-adrenergic agonist that can be taken orally and is useful for prophylaxis. Although β-adrenergic agonists may be delivered orally, adverse effects are minimized when used by inhalation.

192. The answer is d. (*Katzung, pp 336–337.*) The inhibitory effect of mediator release of cromolyn is cell specific. In mast cells exposed to cromolyn, inhibition of the early response occurs to antigen challenge, while in eosinophils, it affects the late response, and in basophils it has almost no effect on mediator release. Cromolyn is effective in antigen-induced asthma, occupation-exposure asthma, and in some cases of intrinsic asthma. Administration of cromolyn by inhalation is most effective in treating patients.

193. The answer is a. (*Hardman, pp 762–764.*) Experimentally, nitrates dilate coronary vessels. This occurs in normal subjects, resulting in an overall increase in coronary blood flow. In arteriosclerotic coronaries, the ability to dilate is lost, and the ischemic area may actually have less blood flow under the influence of nitrates. Improvement in the ischemic conditions is the result of decreased myocardial oxygen demand because of a reduction of preload and afterload. Nitrates dilate both arteries and veins and thereby reduce the work of the heart. Should systemic blood pressure fall, a reflex tachycardia will occur. In pure coronary spasm, such as Prinzmetal's angina, the effect of increased coronary blood flow is relevant, while in severe left ventricular hypertrophy with minimal obstruction, the effect on preload and afterload becomes important.

194. The answer is a. (*Katzung, p 590.*) Bile acids are absorbed primarily in the ileum of the small intestine. Cholestyramine binds bile acids, preventing their reabsorption in the jejunum and ileum. Up to 10-fold greater excretion of bile acids occurs with the use of resins. The increased clearance leads to increased cholesterol turnover of bile acids. Low-density lipoprotein receptor upregulation results in increased uptake of LDL. This does not occur in homozygous familial hypercholesterolemia because of lack of functioning receptors.

195. The answer is c. (*Katzung, p 590.*) Gemfibrozil can interact with the peroxisome proliferator–activated α receptor. Apparently, this leads to an increase in lipolysis of lipoprotein triglyceride by the action on lipoprotein lipase. Although minimal changes occur in plasma LDL levels, there is a decrease in plasma VLDL levels. Plasma HDL cholesterol may increase because of the decreased exchange of triglycerides for cholesteryl esters.

196–197. The answers are 196-b, 197-e. (*Hardman, pp 736, 741, 743–745.*) The enzyme renin acts upon angiotensinogen (an α-globulin) to yield the decapeptide angiotensin I, which has limited pharmacologic activity. Angiotensin I is metabolized extensively in a single passage through the lungs by the carboxypeptidase peptidyl dipeptidase (kinase II, or ACE) to the octapeptide angiotensin II. Angiotensin II has a potent direct action on the vascular smooth muscle and also indirectly stimulates contraction by means of the sympathetic nervous system. The vasoconstriction in response to angiotensin II involves precapillary arterioles and postcapillary venules and results in an increased total peripheral resistance.

Captopril {1-[(25)-3-mercapto-2-methylpropinoyl]-1-proline} is a rationally designed, competitive inhibitor of peptidyl dipeptidase. It blocks the formation but not the response of angiotensin II. Captopril is useful in reducing the blood pressure of both renin-dependent and normal-renin essential hypertension. The hypotensive action of clonidine is believed to be due primarily to stimulation of the α-adrenergic receptors in the CNS. A reduction in the discharge rate of preganglionic adrenergic nerves occurs in addition to bradycardia. The CNS actions of clonidine also lead to a reduction in the level of renin activity in the plasma. Losartan blocks angiotensin type I (AT1) receptors.

198. The answer is d. (*Hardman, pp 885–886. Katzung, pp 591–592.*) Atorvastatin is a structural analogue of an intermediate formed from the action of HMG-CoA reductase. This could result in a modest decrease in plasma cholesterol. Hepatic cholesterol synthesis may decrease significantly; however, nonhepatic tissues increase their rate of synthesis as a compensatory mechanism. The other and perhaps more important effect of the HMG-CoA inhibitors is to increase high-affinity LDL receptors. The plasma LDL is lowered by this action because of an increase in the catabolic rate of LDL and hepatic extraction of LDL precursors.

199. The answer is e. (*Hardman, p 745.*) Vasodilator therapy for CHF has gained prominence in the past 10 years. The ACE inhibitors, such as enalapril, are among the best agents for this purpose, although Ca channel inhibitors and nitroglycerin can also be used. The ACE inhibitors dilate arterioles and veins (reducing preload), as well as inhibit aldosterone production (reducing blood volume), factors considered beneficial in CHF therapy. Both β-adrenergic antagonists and ACE inhibitors have been shown to increase survival in CHF.

200. The answer is c. (*Hardman, pp 774–775.*) β-adrenergic receptor blockers slow heart rate, lower blood pressure, and lessen cardiac contractility without reducing cardiac output; they also have a buffering action against adrenergic stimulation of the cardiac autoregulatory mechanism. These hemodynamic actions decrease the requirement of the heart for oxygen.

201. The answer is d. *(Hardman, p 906.)* Cimetidine slows the metabolism of Ca channel blockers, which are substrates for hepatic mixed-function oxidases. Inhibition of cytochrome P450 activity is peculiar to cimetidine and is not a mechanism of action of other histamine 2 (H_2) blockers.

202. The answer is c. *(Hardman, p 906. Katzung, p 1127.)* Cimetidine inhibits proximal tubular secretion of procainamide, resulting in increased plasma concentrations of procainamide and its active metabolite, N-acetylprocainamide.

203. The answer is b. *(Hardman, pp 816–818.)* Digoxin levels rise with concomitant administration of diltiazem by an unknown mechanism that reduces renal clearance.

204. The answer is d. *(Hardman, pp 816–818.)* Digoxin levels can be reduced by 25% with concomitant use of kaolin-pectin by an unknown mechanism that decreases GI absorption.

Central Nervous System

General anesthetics
Intravenous (IV) anesthetics
Sedatives and hypnotics
Ethanol and related alcohols
Psychotomimetics
Antipsychotics

Antidepressants
Antiepileptics and antiparkinsons
Narcotic analgesics
Local anesthetics
Central nervous system stimulants

Questions

DIRECTIONS: Each item below contains a question or incomplete statement followed by suggested responses. Select the **one best** response to each question.

205. A former heroin addict is maintained on methadone, but succumbs to temptation and buys an opioid on the street. He takes it and rapidly goes into withdrawal. Which opioid did he take?

a. Meperidine
b. Heroin
c. Pentazocine
d. Codeine
e. Propoxyphene

206. Which of the following opioid agonists is only administered by the parenteral route?

a. Morphine
b. Codeine
c. Fentanyl
d. Methadone
e. Propoxyphene

207. Which of the following local anesthetics is useful for topical (surface) administration only?

a. Procaine
b. Bupivacaine
c. Etidocaine
d. Benzocaine
e. Lidocaine

208. Akathisia, Parkinson-like syndrome, galactorrhea, and amenorrhea are side effects of perphenazine, caused by

a. Blockade of muscarinic receptors
b. Blockade of α-adrenergic receptors
c. Blockade of dopamine receptors
d. Supersensitivity of dopamine receptors
e. Stimulation of nicotinic receptors

209. Which of the following agents is useful in the treatment of malignant hyperthermia?

a. Baclofen
b. Diazepam
c. Cyclobenzaprine
d. Dantrolene
e. Halothane

210. Inhibitors of serotonin (5-HT) uptake such as paroxetine interact significantly with which of the following drugs?

a. Chlorpromazine
b. Tranylcypromine
c. Halothane
d. Benztropine
e. Digoxin

211. Which of the following is an antidepressant agent that selectively inhibits serotonin (5-HT) uptake with minimal effect on norepinephrine uptake?

a. Protriptyline
b. Maprotiline
c. Fluoxetine
d. Desipramine
e. Amoxapine

212. Which of the following inhalation anesthetics is most likely to produce hepatotoxicity?

a. Isoflurane
b. Enflurane
c. Methoxyflurane
d. Halothane
e. Nitrous oxide

213. Carbidopa is useful in the treatment of Parkinson's disease because it

a. Is a precursor of levodopa
b. Is a dopaminergic receptor agonist
c. Prevents peripheral biotransformation of L-dopa
d. Prevents a breakdown of dopamine
e. Promotes a decreased concentration of L-dopa in the nigrostriatum

214. Which of the following is described as a competitive benzodiazepine receptor antagonist?

a. Ketamine
b. Chlordiazepoxide
c. Flumazenil
d. Midazolam
e. Triazolam

215. Which one of the following drugs mimics the activity of metenkephalin in the dorsal horn of the spinal cord?

a. Deprenyl (selegiline)
b. Trihexyphenidyl
c. Baclofen
d. Morphine
e. Phenobarbital

216. The preferred treatment of status epilepticus is intravenous administration of

a. Chlorpromazine
b. Diazepam
c. Succinylcholine
d. Tranylcypromine
e. Ethosuximide

217. The most common adverse effect associated with the tricyclic antidepressants is

a. Anticholinergic effects
b. Seizures
c. Arrhythmias
d. Hepatotoxicity
e. Nephrotoxicity

218. A 25-year-old male is seen in the emergency department (ED). He is disoriented but states that he has had nausea, vomiting, abdominal pain, and diarrhea since he took "too many pain pills." Before he can tell you more, he loses consciousness. Liver function tests are abnormal. In addition to gastric lavage, what is the appropriate treatment?

a. Naloxone
b. Diphenoxylate
c. N-acetyl-L-cysteine
d. Prochlorperazine
e. Pralidoxime

219. Which of the following is a selective inhibitor of monoamine oxidase type B (MAO-B) and, therefore, useful in treating parkinsonism?

a. Bromocriptine
b. Carbidopa
c. Selegiline
d. Phenelzine
e. Tranylcypromine

220. Which of the following is associated with abuse of opioid analgesics?

a. No cross-tolerance develops among opioid analgesics
b. Tolerance develops equally to all effects of opioids
c. Opioids reduce pain, aggression, and sexual drives
d. The symptoms of acute methadone withdrawal are qualitatively different from those of acute heroin withdrawal
e. None of the above

221. A 36-year-old male heroin addict is seen in the ED because he cannot be aroused from sleep. On examination, he has shallow breathing and pinpoint pupils. Naloxone is administered, and the patient wakes up. Which of the opiate receptor subtypes that binds naloxone is responsible for reversing the respiratory depression and miosis?

a. δ
b. κ
c. μ

222. A drug that specifically enhances metabolically the activity of brain dopamine is

a. Benztropine
b. Selegiline
c. Trihexyphenidyl
d. Bromocriptine
e. Chlorpromazine

223. A dopamine receptor agonist that is useful in the therapy of Parkinson's disease is

a. Selegiline
b. Bromocriptine
c. Apomorphine
d. Amantidine
e. Belladonna

224. In addition to its use in the treatment of schizophrenia, chlorpromazine is effective

a. In reducing nausea and vomiting
b. As an antihypertensive agent
c. As an antihistaminic
d. In the treatment of depression
e. For treating bipolar affective disorder

225. Morphine may be characterized best by which of the following statements?

a. It is classified as a mixed agonist-antagonist drug
b. It is used medically to inhibit withdrawal symptoms in persons who are dependent on heroin
c. At high doses, it causes death by respiratory depression
d. It is a pure opioid antagonist at the μ, κ, and δ receptors
e. It has an addiction potential equal to that of codeine

226. Cocaine, produced from the leaves of *Erythroxylon* species,

a. Produces bradycardia and vasodilation
b. Is directly related chemically to opioid analgesics
c. Is metabolized by the microsomal metabolizing system
d. Blocks nerve conduction effectively
e. Blocks norepinephrine receptors directly

227. Which of the following agents is a selective dopamine receptor (D_2) agonist?

a. Fluphenazine
b. Bromocriptine
c. Promethazine
d. Haloperidol
e. Chlorpromazine

228. Haloperidol may best be characterized by which of the following statements?

a. It is classified as a phenothiazine
b. It is a selective D_2 receptor agonist
c. Its mechanism of action is completely different from that of chlorpromazine
d. It is more potent as an antipsychotic drug than is chlorpromazine
e. It produces a lower incidence of extrapyramidal reactions than does chlorpromazine

229. A 33-year-old female patient treated with haloperidol for a history of schizophrenia is seen in the ED because of complaints of fever, stiffness, and tremor. Her temperature is 104°F, and her serum creatine kinase (CK) level is elevated. What has occurred?

a. Overdose
b. Allergy
c. Neuroleptic malignant syndrome (NMS)
d. Tardive Dyskinesia
e. Parkinsonism

230. Phencyclidine may best be characterized by which of the following statements?

a. It has opioid activity
b. Its mechanism of action is related to its anticholinergic properties
c. It can cause significant hallucinogenic activity
d. It causes significant withdrawal symptoms
e. Treatment of overdose is with an opiate

231. Which of the following is associated with crack (the free-base form of cocaine)?

a. Flashbacks (recurrences of effects) may occur months after the last use of the drug
b. It may cause seizures and cardiac arrhythmias
c. It acts by blocking adrenergic receptors
d. It is the salt form of cocaine
e. It is primarily administered intranasally

232. In comparing the following neuroleptics, which is most likely to cause marked sedation?

a. Chlorpromazine
b. Haloperidol
c. Resperidone
d. Ziprasidone
e. Sertindole

233. In comparing the following neuroleptics, which is most likely associated with skeletal muscle rigidity, tremor at rest, flat facies, uncontrollable restlessness, and spastic torticollis?

a. Clozapine
b. Haloperidol
c. Olanzapine
d. Sertindole
e. Ziprasidone

234. In comparing the following neuroleptics, which is most likely associated with constipation, urinary retention, blurred vision, and dry mouth?

a. Chlorpromazine
b. Clozapine
c. Olanzapine
d. Sertindole
e. Haloperidol

235. A patient exhibiting multiple facial tics, aggressive outbursts of behavior, and spontaneous repetitive foul language is best treated with which of the following agents?

a. Levodopa
b. Clozapine
c. Thioridazine
d. Haloperidol
e. Trazodone

236. Which of the following may cause nephrogenic diabetes insipidus?

a. Fluoxetine
b. Haloperidol
c. Lithium
d. Phenytoin
e. Diazepam

237. A 36-year-old male with a bipolar disorder is treated with lithium. Among the following adverse effects, which is associated with lithium treatment?

a. Browning of the vision
b. Hypothyroidism
c. Agranulocytosis
d. Neuroleptic malignant syndrome
e. Pseudodepression

238. Which of the following is not associated with the development of a high degree of tolerance following opiate administration?

a. Euphoria
b. Analgesia
c. Nausea and vomiting
d. Respiratory depression
e. Constipation

239. Which of the following is not associated with methadone?

a. It is useful as an analgesic
b. It has greater oral efficacy than morphine
c. It possesses opioid antagonist effects
d. It produces a milder but more protracted withdrawal syndrome than that associated with morphine
e. Adverse reactions may include constipation, respiratory depression, and lightheadedness

240. A 40-year-old male with repetitive obsessive behavior that prevents him from carrying out simple tasks is treated with fluoxetine. How is fluoxetine classified?

a. As an MAO inhibitor (MAOI)
b. As a tricyclic nonselective amine reuptake inhibitor
c. As a heterocyclic nonselective amine reuptake inhibitor
d. As a selective serotonin reuptake inhibitor
e. As an α_2-adrenergic receptor inhibitor
f. As a muscarinic receptor inhibitor

241. Which of the following is not associated with the ingestion of ethanol?

a. It is a hepatotoxic agent
b. It elevates body temperature
c. It suppresses the release of antidiuretic hormone
d. It can lead to gastritis and pancreatitis
e. Acute overdose can cause acidosis, hypoglycemia, and elevated intracranial pressure

242. A 25-year-old male with difficulty sleeping and poor appetite associated with weight loss is placed on amitriptyline. How is amitriptyline classified?

a. As an MAOI
b. As a tricyclic nonselective amine reuptake inhibitor
c. As a heterocyclic nonselective amine reuptake inhibitor
d. As a selective serotonin reuptake inhibitor
e. As an α_2-adrenergic receptor inhibitor
f. As a muscarinic receptor inhibitor

243. A patient with intractable itching would best respond to which of the following?

a. Chlorpromazine
b. Pimozide
c. Haloperidol
d. Risperidone
e. Clozapine

244. Which of the following antipsychotics requires weekly blood counts?

a. Chlorpromazine
b. Clozapine
c. Haloperidol
d. Olanzapine
e. Molindone

245. Which of the following is not associated with enhancement of the activity of γ-aminobutyric acid (GABA)

a. Chlordiazepoxide
b. Phenobarbital
c. Diazepam
d. Valproic acid
e. Chlorpromazine

246. Which of the following is not characterisitic of marijuana?

a. It may lower intraocular pressure
b. A sign of acute intoxication is reddening of conjunctiva
c. It has antiemetic properties
d. Heavy chronic use can lower serum testosterone levels in men
e. It causes flashbacks

247. Which of the following agents is effective in minimizing emotional bluntness and social withdrawal seen in schizophrenia?

a. Chlorpromazine
b. Haloperidol
c. Olanzapine
d. Fluphenazine
e. Thiothixene

248. A 26-year-old female with reactive depression complains of missing her period and having milk discharge from her breasts. She has no signs of pregnancy, including a negative pregnancy test. Which of the following might have caused these findings?

a. Clomipramine
b. Amoxapine
c. Fluoxetine
d. Mirtazapine
e. Tranylcypromine

249. Which of the following does not produce its pharmacologic effects by inhibition of prostaglandin synthesis?

a. Indomethacin
b. Ibuprofen
c. Acetaminophen
d. Piroxicam
e. Naproxen

250. With increasing concentrations of a local anesthetic, the order of effect is

a. Pain fibers—sensory fibers—motor fibers
b. Sensory fibers—pain fibers—motor fibers
c. Pain fibers—motor fibers—sensory fibers
d. Sensory fibers—motor fibers—pain fibers
e. Motor fibers—sensory fibers—pain fibers
f. Motor fibers—pain fibers—sensory fibers
g. Pain fibers—sensory fibers—no effect on motor fibers
h. Sensory fibers—pain fibers—no effect on motor fibers

251. A 55-year-old female given a general anesthetic for a surgical procedure develops hyperthermia, hypertension, hyperkalemia, tachycardia, muscle rigidity, and metabolic acidosis. Which of the following general anesthetics did she receive?

a. Ketamine
b. Midazolam
c. Thiopental
d. Propofol
e. Halothane

252. A 20-year-old female with a history of grand mal seizures who is well controlled on seizure medication complains of losing her balance. Which of the following agents could account for this adverse effect?

a. Primidone
b. Disulfiram
c. Dextroamphetamine
d. Valproic acid
e. Flurazepam
f. Phenylephrine
g. Phenytoin
h. Isoetharine
i. Carbamazepine
j. Amitriptyline
k. Triazolam
l. Diazepam

253. A 30-year-old alcoholic with no apparent liver disease has decided to abstain from alcohol. Shortly thereafter, he becomes agitated, anxious, has visual hallucinations, is generally totally disoriented, and suffers bouts of insomnia. Which of the following agents might be of use in averting these findings?

a. Primidone
b. Disulfiram
c. Dextroamphetamine
d. Valproic acid
e. Phenylephrine
f. Phenytoin
g. Isoetharine
h. Carbamazepine
i. Amitriptyline
j. Triazolam
k. Diazepam

254. Although a patient was instructed not to use alcohol because of a medication he was taking, he did not listen to advice and decided to have a drink of alcohol. Within minutes, he developed flushing, a throbbing headache, nausea and vomiting. Which of the following medications was he taking?

a. Naltrexone
b. Diazepam
c. Disulfiram
d. Phenobarbital
e. Tranylcypromine

255. At a follow-up visit one month after a 22-year-old male was newly diagnosed with schizophrenia and started on chlorpromazine, he has several complaints, listed below. Which of the following cannot be attributed to chlorpromazine?

a. Restless feeling
b. Sexual dysfunction
c. Urinary hesitancy
d. Vomiting

256. A 27-year-old male presents with reactive depression following the accidental death of a close relative. A tricyclic antidepressant is chosen to control his depression. Which adverse effect would not be of concern?

a. Disturbance in rapid-eye-movement (REM) sleep
b. Sedation
c. Dry mouth
d. Orthostatic hypotension
e. Tardive dyskinesia

DIRECTIONS: Each group of questions below consists of lettered options followed by a set of numbered items. For each numbered item, select the **one** lettered option with which it is **most** closely associated. Each lettered option may be used once, more than once, or not at all.

Questions 257–260

For each patient, select the drug of choice:

a. Midazolam
b. Diazepam
c. Alprazolam
d. Ethosuximide
e. Oxazepam

257. A 38-year-old male with a 15-year history of grand mal seizures is brought to the ED with generalized tonic-clonic seizures that are unremittent.

258. A 16-year-old female is brought to the ED by her mother, who has observed that her daughter has abruptly experienced an impairment of consciousness associated with clonic jerking of the eyelids and staring into space lasting approximately 30 s.

259. A 48-year-old female has had difficulty swallowing for six months. She is premedicated for an endoscopic examination.

260. A 12-year-old boy develops uncontrollable panic while camping with his parents in the Mojave Desert.

261. A 20-year-old male with absence seizures is treated with ethosuximide. What is the principal mechanism of action of ethosuximide?

a. Sodium channel blockade
b. Increase in the frequency of the chloride channel opening
c. Increase in GABA
d. Calcium channel blockade
e. Increased potassium channel permeability
f. NMDA receptor blockade

262. A 30-year-old female with partial seizures is treated with vigabatrin. What is the principal mechanism of action of vigabatrin?

a. Sodium channel blockade
b. Increase in frequency of chloride channel opening
c. Increase in GABA
d. Calcium channel blockade
e. Increased potassium channel permeability
f. NMDA receptor blockade

263. Of the following antiepileptic agents, which is associated with causing psychosis?

a. Phenobarbital
b. Ethosuximide
c. Phenytoin
d. Vigabatrin
e. Valproic acid

Questions 264–265

For each of the drugs listed below, choose the effect that it usually produces.

a. Tachyphylaxis
b. Physical dependence only
c. Tolerance and physical dependence
d. Hallucinations
e. Psychedelic effects
f. Low potential of addiction

264. Meperidine

265. Secobarbital

266. A pediatric patient treated for grand mal seizures develops abnormal values on liver function tests. Which of the following antiepileptic agents would cause this to occur?

a. Carbamezine
b. Valproic acid
c. Phenytoin
d. Phenobarbital
e. Gabapentin

267. A 19-year-old female whose roommate is being treated for depression decides that she is also depressed and secretly takes her roommate's pills "as directed on the bottle" for several days. One night, she makes herself a snack of chicken liver paté and bleu cheese, accompanied by a glass of red wine. She soon develops headache, nausea, and palpitations. She goes to the ED, where her blood pressure is found to be 200/110 mmHg. What antidepressant did she take?

a. Sertraline
b. Phenelzine
c. Nortriptyline
d. Trazodone
e. Fluoxetine

268. A 41-year-old female is seen in the psychiatric clinic for a follow-up appointment. She has been taking an antidepressant for three weeks with some improvement in mood. However, she complains of drowsiness, palpitations, dry mouth, and feeling faint on standing. Which antidepressant is she taking?

a. Amitriptyline
b. Trazodone
c. Fluoxetine
d. Venlafaxine
e. Bupropion

269. A 31-year-old female has been treated with fluoxetine for two months with no improvement in her depression. You decide to switch antidepressant therapy to phenelzine and instruct her to wait one week after stopping fluoxetine to start taking the new pills. She begins therapy immediately with phenyline without discontinuing fluoxetine. Two days later, she is brought to the ED with unstable vital signs, muscle rigidity, myoclonus, and hyperthermia. What caused these findings?

a. Increased serotonin (5-HT) in synapses
b. Increased norepinephrine in synapses
c. Increased acetylcholine in synapses
d. Increased dopamine in synapses

270. A 36-year-old male unemployed dishwasher with no history of seizures presents with difficulty thinking coherently and claims that he is an astronaut. Following treatment, he suddenly has a grand mal seizure. Which neuroleptic agent was administered?

a. Haloperidol
b. Fluphenazine
c. Clozapine
d. Molindone
e. Loxapine

271. A 31-year-old female is treated with an antipsychotic agent because of a recent history of spontaneously removing her clothing in public places and claiming that she hears voices telling her to do so. Her blood pressure is normally 130/70 mmHg. Since being treated with a drug, she has had several bouts of syncope. Orthostatic hypotension was noted on physical examination. Which drug most likely caused this?

a. Haloperidol
b. Olanzapine
c. Fluphenazine
d. Chlorpromazine
e. Sertindole

272. A 29-year-old male uses secobarbital to satisfy his addiction to barbiturates. During the past week, he is imprisoned and is not able to obtain the drug. He is brought to the prison medical ward because of the onset of severe anxiety, increased sensitivity to light, dizziness, and generalized tremors. On physical examination, he is hyperreflexic. Which of the following agents should he be given to diminish his withdrawal symptoms?

a. Buspirone
b. Chloral hydrate
c. Chlorpromazine
d. Diazepam
e. Trazodone

273. A 72-year-old female with a long history of anxiety treated with diazepam decides to triple her dose because of increasing fearfulness about "environmental noises." Several days after her attempt at self-prescribing, her neighbor finds her to be extremely lethargic and nonresponsive. On examination, she is found to be stuporous and have diminished reaction to pain and decreased reflexes. Her respiratory rate is 8 breaths per minute (BPM), and she has shallow respirations. Which antidote could be given to reverse these findings?

a. Naltrexone
b. Physostigmine
c. Pralidoxime
d. Flumazenil

274. A 36-year-old male has been experiencing intense pressure to be more productive at work. This has resulted in his becoming extremely anxious, which makes it very difficult for him to function effectively. He wishes to keep his job. Physical examination and blood chemistries are normal. He is given diazepam, which diminishes his anxiety and allows him to concentrate on his work. What is the mechanism of action of diazepam?

a. It directly opens the Cl^- channel of the GABA receptor
b. It increases the frequency of opening of the Cl^- channel of the GABA receptor
c. It prolongs the duration of opening of the Cl^- channel of the GABA receptor

275. Neural tube defects may occur with which of the following anti-seizure drugs?

a. Ethosuximide
b. Vigabratin
c. Phenobarbital
d. Valproic acid
e. Primidone

276. A 29-year-old male requires suturing for a deep laceration in his palm. He is allergic to benzocaine. Which of the following local anesthetics could safely be used?

a. Cocaine
b. Tetracaine
c. Bupivacaine
d. Procaine

277. A 45-year-old male with alcoholic cirrhosis is seen in the ED because of a laceration of the scalp. Of the following local anesthetics, which would potentially be toxic?

a. Lidocaine
b. Benzocaine
c. Procaine
d. Tetracaine

278. Which best describes the mechanism of interaction of cimetidine with benzodiazepine?

a. It decreases benzodiazepine's metabolism
b. It decreases benzodiazepine's sensitivity at the site of action
c. It decreases benzodiazepine's renal excretion
d. It decreases benzodiazepine's plasma protein binding
e. It decreases benzodiazepine's intestinal absorption

279. Which best describes the mechanism of interaction of nonsteroidal anti-inflammatory drugs (NSAIDs) with lithium salts?

a. They increase lithium intestinal absorption
b. They increase lithium renal reabsorption
c. They increase lithium plasma protein binding
d. They increase lithium sensitivity at its site of action

Central Nervous System

Answers

205. The answer is c. (*Hardman, p 546.*) Pentazocine is a mixed agonist-antagonist of opioid receptors. When a partial agonist, such as pentazocine, displaces a full agonist, such as methadone, the receptor is less activated; this leads to withdrawal syndrome in an opioid-dependent person.

206. The answer is c. (*Hardman, pp 543–544. Katzung, p 253.*) Fentanyl is a chemical relative of meperidine that is nearly 100 times more potent than morphine. The duration of action, usually between 30 and 60 min after parenteral administration, is shorter than that of meperidine. Fentanyl citrate is only available for parenteral administration intramuscularly and intravenously. Transbuccal ("lollipop") and transdermal patches avoid first-pass metabolism of fentanyl.

207. The answer is d. (*Katzung, p 437.*) Local anesthetics are agents that, when applied locally, block nerve conduction; they also prevent generation of a nerve impulse. All contain a lipophilic (benzene) functional group and most a hydrophilic (amine) group. Benzocaine does not contain the terminal hydrophilic amine group; thus, it is only slightly soluble in water and is slowly absorbed with a prolonged duration. It is, therefore, only useful as a surface anesthetic.

208. The answer is c. (*Hardman, pp 414–416.*) Unwanted pharmacologic side effects produced by phenothiazine antipsychotic drugs (e.g., perphenazine) include Parkinson-like syndrome, akathisia, dystonias, galactorrhea, amenorrhea, and infertility. These side effects are due to the ability of these agents to block dopamine receptors. The phenothiazines also block muscarinic and α-adrenergic receptors, which are responsible for other effects.

209. The answer is d. (*Hardman, p 188.*) Malignant hyperthermia (hyperpyrexia), a syndrome that is associated with the use of a general anesthetic (e.g., halothane) in conjunction with a skeletal muscle relaxant, is characterized by tachycardia, hyperventilation, arrhythmias, fever, muscular fasciculation, and rigidity. It is caused by a sudden increase in the availability of calcium (Ca) ions in the myoplasma of muscle. Dantrolene, which interferes with release of Ca ions from the sarcoplasmic reticulum, is indicated in treatment of the disorder. The first three agents are centrally acting skeletal muscle relaxants that are not useful in the treatment of malignant hyperthermia.

210. The answer is b. *(Katzung, p 1130.)* Fatalities have been reported when fluoxetine and MAO inhibitors (MAOIs) such as tranylcypromine have been given simultaneously. The MAOIs should be stopped at least two weeks before the administration of fluoxetine or paroxetine. The mechanism of this interaction is under investigation.

211. The answer is c. *(Hardman, p 436.)* The tricyclics and second-generation antidepressants act by blocking serotonin or norepinephrine uptake into the presynaptic terminal. Fluoxetine selectively inhibits serotonin uptake with minimal effects on norepinephrine uptake. Protriptyline, maprotiline, desipramine, and amoxapine have greater effect on norepinephrine uptake.

212. The answer is d. *(Hardman, pp 308–313.)* Halothane is a substituted alkane general anesthetic. It undergoes significant metabolism in humans with about 20% of the absorbed dose recovered as metabolites. Halothane can cause postoperative jaundice and hepatic necrosis with repeated administration in rare instances.

213. The answer is c. *(Hardman, p 510.)* Carbidopa is an inhibitor of aromatic L-amino acid decarboxylase. It cannot readily penetrate the central nervous system (CNS) and, thus, decreases the decarboxylation of L-dopa in the peripheral tissues. This promotes an increased concentration of L-dopa in the nigrostriatum, where it is converted to dopamine. In addition, the effective dose of L-dopa can be reduced.

214. The answer is c. *(Katzung, pp 373–374.)* Flumazenil is a competitive benzodiazepine receptor antagonist. The drug reverses the CNS sedative effects of benzodiazepines and is indicated where general anesthesia has been induced by or maintained with benzodiazepines such as diazepam, lorazepam, or midazolam.

215. The answer is d. *(Hardman, pp 521–522.)* The enkephalins are endogenous agonists of the opioid receptors. They are located in areas of the brain and spinal cord related to the perception of pain. These areas include the laminae I and II of the spinal cord, the spinal trigeminal nucleus, and the periaqueductal gray. Selegiline and trihexyphenidyl are anti-Parkinsonism drugs; baclofen is a skeletal muscle relaxant agonist for the GABA receptor.

216. The answer is b. *(Hardman, p 484.)* Intravenously administered diazepam is the drug of choice for treatment of status epilepticus. Diazepam increases the apparent affinity of the inhibitory neurotransmitter GABA for binding sites on brain cell membranes. The effects of diazepam are short-lasting. Continuing therapy is usually with phenytoin. Other drugs suggested for use in status epilepticus are lorazepam and lidocaine. None of the other drugs listed in the question are appropriate for status epilepticus: chlorpromazine is an antipsychotic; succinylcholine is a neuromuscular blocking agent; tranylcypromine is an antidepressant; ethosuximide is used in petit mal epilepsy.

217. The answer is a. *(Hardman, p 436.)* The most common side effects associated with tricyclic antidepressants are their antimuscarinic effects, which may be evident in over 50% of patients. Clinically, the antimuscarinic effects may manifest as dry mouth, blurred vision, constipation, tachycardia, dizziness, and urinary retention. At therapeutic plasma concentrations, these drugs usually do not cause changes in the EKG. Direct cardiac effects of the tricyclic antidepressants are important in overdosage.

218. The answer is c. *(Hardman, pp 632–633.)* Nausea, vomiting, abdominal pain, and diarrhea are early signs of the severe liver toxicity caused by high levels of acetaminophen; other symptoms of acetaminophen toxicity include dizziness, excitement, and disorientation. N-acetyl-L-cysteine is the appropriate treatment for acetaminophen overdose.

219. The answer is c. *(Katzung, pp 469–470.)* Two types of MAO have been found: (1) MAO-A, which metabolizes norepinephrine and serotonin, and (2) MAO-B, which metabolizes dopamine. Selegiline is a selective inhibitor of MAO-B. It therefore inhibits the breakdown of dopamine and prolongs the therapeutic effectiveness of L-dopa in parkinsonism. Bromocriptine is a dopamine receptor agonist. Carbidopa inhibits the peripheral metabolism of L-dopa. Both are useful in the treatment of parkinsonism. Phenelzine and tranylcypromine are nonselective MAOIs. Combining them with L-dopa may lead to hypertensive crises, and thus they are not used in the therapy of parkinsonism.

220. The answer is c. *(Hardman, pp 556–559.)* In opioid abuse, there is always a high degree of cross-tolerance to other drugs with a similar pharmacologic action even if the chemical composition of the opioids is totally different. Tolerance develops at different rates to different effects of opioids. With methadone, abrupt withdrawal causes a syndrome that is qualitatively similar to that of morphine but is longer and less intense, thus following the general rule that a drug with a shorter duration of action produces a shorter, more intense withdrawal syndrome. The crimes associated with narcotic abuse are considered to be motivated by the need to acquire the drug and not from the effects of the drug per se. Significant tolerance develops to most of the effects of narcotics, except for constipation and pinpoint pupils, to which there is minimal tolerance.

221. The answer is c. *(Hardman, p 527. Katzung, p 516.)* Naloxone is a pure opioid antagonist at the μ, κ, and δ receptors. μ-receptor stimulation causes analgesia, euphoria, decreased gastrointestinal (GI) activity, miosis, and respiratory depression. κ-receptor stimulation causes analgesia, dysphoria, and psychotomimetic effects. δ-receptor stimulation is not fully understood in humans, but is associated with analgesia and antinociception for thermal stimuli.

222. The answer is b. *(Hardman, p 451.)* Selegiline inhibits MAO-B, thus delaying the metabolic breakdown of dopamine. It is effective alone in parkinsonism and increases the effectiveness of L-dopa. Benztropine and trihexyphenidyl are cholinergic antagonists in the brain; bromocriptine is a dopamine receptor agonist. Chlorpromazine is an antipsychotic drug with antiadrenergic properties.

223. The answer is b. *(Katzung, pp 468–469.)* Bromocriptine mimics the action of dopamine in the brain but is not as readily metabolized. It is especially useful in parkinsonism that is unresponsive to L-dopa. Apomorphine is also a dopamine receptor agonist, but its side effects preclude its use for this purpose. Selegiline is an MAO-B inhibitor, atropine is a belladonna preparation, and amantadine is an antiviral agent that probably affects the synthesis or uptake of dopamine.

224. The answer is a. (*Hardman, pp 418–419, 930.*) Chlorpromazine is the prototype compound of the phenothiazine class of antipsychotic drugs. It is indicated for use in the treatment of a variety of psychoses, which includes schizophrenia, and in the treatment of nausea and vomiting, in both adults and children, from a number of causes. The drug can be administered orally, rectally, or intramuscularly for this purpose. It is believed that the effectiveness of the compound is based on the inhibition of dopaminergic receptors in the chemoreceptor trigger zone of the medulla. Other phenothiazine derivatives are also used for emesis, including thiethylperazine, prochlorperazine, and perphenazine. Although chlorpromazine may cause orthostatic hypotension and has mild H_1-histamine receptor blocking activity, the drug is never used as an antihypertensive or as an antihistaminic. Chlorpromazine is not an effective antidepressant drug, and lithium salts are used for treating the mania that is associated with bipolar affective disorder.

225. The answer is c. (*Hardman, pp 528–537.*) Morphine is a pure agonist opioid drug with agonist activity toward all the opioid subtype receptor sites. In high doses, deaths associated with morphine are related to the depression of the respiratory center in the medulla. Morphine has a high addiction potential related to the activity of heroin or dihydromorphine. Codeine has a significantly lower addiction potential.

226. The answer is d. (*Hardman, pp 338, 570.*) Cocaine has local anesthetic properties; it can block the initiation or conduction of a nerve impulse. It is biotransformed by plasma esterases to inactive products. In addition, cocaine blocks the reuptake of norepinephrine. This action produces CNS stimulant effects including euphoria, excitement, and restlessness. Peripherally, cocaine produces sympathomimetic effects including tachycardia and vasoconstriction. Death from acute overdose can be from respiratory depression or cardiac failure. Cocaine is an ester of benzoic acid and is closely related to the structure of atropine.

227. The answer is b. (*Hardman, pp 282–283.*) Central dopamine receptors are divided into D_1 and D_2 receptors. Antipsychotic activity is better correlated to blockade of D_2 receptors. Haloperidol, a potent antipsychotic, selectively antagonizes at D_2 receptors. Phenothiazine derivatives, such as chlorpromazine, fluphenazine, and promethazine, are not selective for D_2 receptors. Bromocriptine, a selective D_2 agonist, is useful in the treatment of parkinsonism and hyperprolactinemia. It produces fewer adverse reactions than do nonselective dopamine receptor agonists.

228. The answer is d. (*Hardman, pp 407–412.*) Haloperidol is a butyrophenone derivative with the same mechanism of action as the phenothiazines, that is, blockade of dopaminergic receptors. It is more selective for D_2 receptors. Haloperidol is more potent on a weight basis than the phenothiazines, but produces a higher incidence of extrapyramidal reactions than does chlorpromazine.

229. The answer is c. (*Hardman, pp 415–416.*) Neuroleptic malignant syndrome is thought to be a severe form of an extrapyramidal syndrome that can occur at any time with any dose of a neuroleptic agent. However, the risk is higher when high-potency agents are used in high doses, especially if given parenterally. Mortality from NMS is greater than 10%.

230. The answer is c. (*Hardman, pp 574–575.*) Phencyclidine is a hallucinogenic compound with no opioid activity. Its mechanism of action is amphetamine-like. A withdrawal syndrome has not been described for this drug in human subjects. In overdose, the treatment of choice for the psychotic activity is the antipsychotic drug haloperidol.

231. The answer is b. (*Katzung, p 538.*) Crack is the free-base (nonsalt) form of the alkaloid cocaine. It is called *crack* because, when heated, it makes a crackling sound. Heating crack enables a person to smoke it; the drug is readily absorbed through the lungs and produces an intense euphoric effect in seconds. Use has led to seizures and cardiac arrhythmias. Some of cocaine's effects (sympathomimetic) are due to blockade of norepinephrine reuptake into presynaptic terminals; it does not block receptors. *Flashbacks* can occur with use of LSD and mescaline but have not been associated with the use of cocaine.

232. The answer is a. *(Katzung, p 482.)* Phenothiazines as a class and, in particular, the aliphatic phenothiazines are most likely to produce marked sedation. The mechanism of action for this effect is associated with its ability to block histamine and acetylcholine receptors.

233. The answer is b. *(Katzung, p 482.)* Haloperidol, a butyrophenone, is by far the most likely antipsychotic to produce extrapyramidal toxicities. Other agents, such as piperazine (an aromatic phenothiazine), thiothixene (a thioxanthene), and pimozide (a diphenylbutyropiperidine) are comparitively less likely to produce extrapyramidal toxicity than haloperidol. The antagonism of dopamine in the nigrostriatal system might explain the Parkinson-like effects. Both haloperidol and pimozide act mainly on D_2 receptors, whereas thioridazine and piperazine act on α-adrenergic receptors, and have a less potent but definite effect on D_2 receptors.

234. The answer is a. *(Katzung, pp 471, 473, 482.)* The phenothiazines as a class are the most potent anticholinergics of the neuroleptics. Tolerance to their anticholinergic effects occurs in most patients. Cholinomimetic agents may be used to overcome symptoms that persist.

235. The answer is d. *(Hardman, p 420. Katzung, p 485.)* Tourette's syndrome is effectively treated with haloperidol, a high-potency antipsychotic. If patients are unresponsive or do not tolerate haloperidol, they might be switched to pimozide.

236. The answer is c. *(Katzung, p 493.)* Lithium treatment frequently causes polyuria and polydipsia. The collecting tubule of the kidney loses the capacity to conserve water via antidiuretic hormone. This results in significant free-water clearance, which is referred to as *nephrogenic diabetes insipidus.*

237. The answer is b. *(Katzung, pp 493–494.)* A decrease in thyroid function occurs in most patients on lithium. This effect is usually reversible or not progressive, but a few patients develop symptoms of hypothyroidism. A serum thyroid-stimulating hormone (TSH) concentration is recommended every 6 to 12 months. "Browning" of vision, clinically described as *pigmentary retinopathy,* occurs with thioridazine. This is due to retinal deposition of the drug. Although neurologic adverse effects (e.g., tremor, choreoathetosis, motor hyperactivity, ataxia, dysarthria, and aphasia) can occur with lithium, it does not cause the neuroleptic malignant syndrome associated with antipsychotic agents. *Pseudodepression* sometimes occurs in patients on antipsychotics. This may be related to drug-induced akinesia.

238. The answer is e. *(Hardman, pp 528–537.)* The extent and rate at which tolerance develops to the effects of opioid analgesics vary. A high degree of tolerance develops to analgesia, euphoria, sedation, respiratory depression, antidiuresis, nausea and vomiting, and cough suppression. A moderate degree develops to bradycardia. Little or no tolerance develops to the drug-induced miosis, constipation, and convulsions.

239. The answer is c. *(Hardman, pp 544–545.)* Methadone is an opioid receptor agonist. It is used as an analgesic and to treat opioid abstinence and heroin users (methadone maintenance). The drug has greater oral efficacy than morphine and a much longer biologic half-life; this accounts for the milder but more protracted abstinence syndrome associated with methadone. Methadone does not possess opioid antagonist properties and, thus, would not precipitate withdrawal symptoms in a heroin addict, as would naloxone or naltrexone.

240. The answer is d. *(Katzung, p 505.)* Fluoxetine is a highly selective serotonin reuptake inhibitor (SSRI) acting on the 5-HT transporter. It forms an active metabolite that is effective for several days. Selective serotonin reuptake inhibitors are inhibitors of cytochrome P450 isoenzymes, which is the basis of potential drug-drug interactions.

241. The answer is b. *(Hardman, pp 386–393.)* Ethanol is a CNS depressant. Among its many effects, it suppresses the release of antidiuretic hormone. Ethanol also causes peripheral vasodilation, particularly of cutaneous blood vessels. Though this may give one a feeling of warmth, heat is being dissipated and body temperature lowered. Chronic use can lead to gastritis, pancreatitis, cirrhosis of the liver, and central effects such as Wernicke's encephalopathy and Korsakoff's psychosis. Acute overdose can lead to acidosis, hypoglycemia, and elevated intracranial pressure.

242. The answer is b. *(Katzung, p 499. Hardman, p 433.)* Amitriptyline is a tertiary amine tricyclic antidepressant. It functions as a norepinephrine reuptake inhibitor. Brain levels of amines are increased. This results in increased vesicular stores of norepinephrine and serotonin. Amitriptyline is a prototypical tricyclic antidepressant that has proved useful in patients with sleep and appetite disorders.

243. The answer is a. *(Katzung, p 485.)* Agents with H_1 receptor blocking actions are effective in reducing itching. H_1 receptor blockade is typical of phenothiazines with short side chains.

244. The answer is b. *(Katzung, p 486.)* Clozapine causes agranulocytosis in 1% to 2% of treated patients. It is generally reversible on discontinuation of the drug. Weekly blood tests are recommended for patients who are treated with clozapine. Agranulocytosis occurs rarely with other high-potency antipsychotic agents.

245. The answer is e. *(Hardman, pp 280–281.)* γ-aminobutyric acid is an inhibitory neurotransmitter that activates the Cl^- channel. Benzodiazepines (e.g., chlordiazepoxide, diazepam) bind to receptors on the Cl^- channel and enhance the binding of GABA to its receptor. Barbiturates also act on the Cl^- channel to increase the opening frequency of the channel. Valproic acid elevates brain levels of GABA by inhibiting GABA metabolism. Chlorpromazine blocks the activity of dopamine receptors and has little or no effect on the GABA system.

246. The answer is e. *(Hardman, pp 572–573.)* The active ingredient in marijuana is Δ-9-tetrahydrocannabinol. In general, marijuana is a CNS stimulant causing tachycardia, giddiness, and, at high doses, visual hallucinations. Acute intoxication is characterized by reddening of the conjunctiva (bloodshot eyes) owing to local vasodilation. Potential therapeutic uses include antiemesis in cancer chemotherapy and reduction of intraocular pressure in glaucoma. Chronic use has been associated with an amotivational syndrome and with a reduction in serum testosterone and sperm count. Flashbacks are a major symptom of LSD use.

247. The answer is c. *(Katzung, pp 485–486.)* In addition to its antipsychotic action, olanzapine diminishes emotional bluntness and social withdrawl that are seen in schizophrenic patients, without significant anticholinergic and extrapyramidal effects.

248. The answer is b. *(Katzung, pp 504–505.)* Amoxapine is a heterocyclic antidepressant that has effects on norepinephrine and serotonin uptake. It is useful in psychotic patients who are depressed. The dopaminergic antagonism caused by amoxapine may lead to the amenorrhea-galactorrhea syndrome.

249. The answer is c. *(Hardman, pp 617–642.)* All of the drugs mentioned, with the exception of acetaminophen, achieve their therapeutic and toxic effects by inhibition of prostaglandin synthesis. Known as NSAIDs, the group includes salicylates as well as sulindac and fenoprofen. Acetaminophen is equal in analgesic potency to NSAIDS, but has no effect on prostaglandins. It is also nonulcerogenic—a great advantage in patients who are ulcer-prone.

250. The answer is a. *(Katzung, pp 439–441.)* The primary effect of local anesthetics is blockade of voltage channel–gated Na channels. Progressively increasing concentrations of local anesthetics results in an increased threshold of excitation, a slowing of impulse conduction, a decline in the rate of rise of the action potential, a decrease in the height of the action potential, and eventual obliteration of the action potential. Local anesthetics first block small unmyelinated or lightly myelinated fibers (pain), followed by heavily myelinated but small-diameter fibers (sensory) and then larger-diameter fibers (proprioception, pressure, motor).

251. The answer is e. *(Katzung, pp 428–429.)* Although a rare occurrence, halothane and other inhaled gas anesthetics may cause malignant hyperthermia. Apparently, this occurs in genetically susceptible individuals. Its onset may be accelerated by the concomitant use of succinylcholine. Immediate treatment includes administration of dantrolene.

252. The answer is g. *(Katzung, pp 399–400.)* Phenytoin is one of the most commonly used antiepileptic agents. Chronic administration has been reported to cause adverse reactions, such as ataxia, dizziness, nystagmus, gingival hyperplasia, hirsutism, and megaloblastic anemia.

253. The answer is k. *(Katzung, p 390.)* Long-acting benzodiazepams such as diazepam are useful in alcohol withdrawal. Its active metabolite is eliminated slowly, thereby increasing its duration of action. In patients with liver disease, short-acting agents might prove effective if they are metabolized to inactive water-soluble metabolites (e.g., oxazepam). Triazolam would be useful because of its short duration of action.

254. The answer is c. *(Katzung, pp 390–391.)* Disulfiram is used in controlling alcohol consumption. The onset of symptoms is almost immediately following ingestion of alcohol and may last for several hours in some patients. Disulfiram acts by inhibition of aldehyde dehydrogenase, resulting in the accumulation of acetaldehyde. Central nervous system depression can occur with centrally acting sedative agents such as diazepam and phenobarbital.

255. The answer is d. *(Hardman, p 414.)* Antipsychotic agents, particularly prochlorperazine, are also useful as antiemetic agents, thought to be due to dopamine blockade at the stomach and at the chemoreceptor trigger zone of the medulla.

256. The answer is e. *(Hardman, pp 415, 442–443.)* Tardive dyskinesia is an adverse effect of neuroleptics, not tricyclic, antidepressants.

257. The answer is b. *(Hardman, p 484. Katzung, p 415.)* Intravenous diazepam given immediately is highly effective in controlling status epilepticus.

258. The answer is d. *(Katzung, p 408.)* Ethosuximide is very effective in absence seizures. Clonazepam is also effective.

259. The answer is a. *(Hardman, p 373. Katzung, pp 430–431.)* Midazolam is useful for sedation because it produces a higher incidence of amnesia and has a more rapid onset of action and a shorter half-life than other benzodiazepines used in anesthesia.

260. The answer is c. *(Hardman, p 372. Katzung, p 375.)* Compared with other benzodiazepines, alprazolam is selective for treating agoraphobia and panic disorders.

261. The answer is d. *(Katzung, pp 408–409.)* Ethosuximide is especially useful in the treatment of absence seizures. Although it may act at several sites, the principal mechanism of action is on T-type Ca currents in thalamic neurons at relevant concentrations. This action blocks the pacemaker current that effects the generation of rhythmic cortical discharge associated with an absence attack.

262. The answer is c. *(Hardman, p 481. Katzung, pp 404–405.)* Vigabatrin is useful in partial seizures. It is an irreversible inhibitor of GABA aminotransferase, an enzyme responsible for the termination of GABA action. This results in accumulation of GABA at synaptic sites, thereby enhancing its effect.

263. The answer is d. *(Katzung, pp 404–405.)* Vigabatrin can induce psychosis. It is recommended that it not be used in patients with preexisting depression and psychosis.

264–265. The answers are 264-c, 265-c. *(Katzung, pp 519, 535–537.)* Heroin and other opioids (such as morphine and meperidine) exhibit a high degree of tolerance and physical dependence. The tolerance rate magnitudes to all of the effects of opioids are not necessarily the same. The physical dependence is quite clear from the character and severity of withdrawal symptoms, which include vomiting spasms, abdominal cramps, diarrhea, and acid-base imbalances among others.

Secobarbital exhibits the same pharmacologic properties as other members of the barbiturate class. Most nonmedical use is with short-acting barbiturates, such as secobarbital. Although there may be considerable tolerance to the sedative and intoxicating effects of the drug, the lethal dose is not much greater in addicted than in normal persons. Tolerance does not develop to the respiratory effect. The combination of alcohol and barbiturates may lead to fatalities because of their combined respiratory depressive effects. Similar outcomes may occur with the benzodiazepines. Severe withdrawal symptoms in epileptic patients may include grand mal seizures and delirium.

266. The answer is b. *(Katzung, p 411.)* Severe hepatotoxicity of an idiosyncratic nature is associated with valproic acid. The risk is very high in the pediatric population, particularly in patients below the age of two. Fatalities generally occur within four months of treatment. Hepatotoxicity may be reversed in some individuals.

267. The answer is b. (*Hardman, p 444.*) This patient ate tyramine-rich foods while taking an MAOI and went into hypertensive crisis. Tyramine causes release of stored catecholamines from presynaptic terminals, which can cause hypertension, headache, tachycardia, cardiac arrhythmias, nausea, and stroke. In patients who do not take MAOIs, tyramine is inactivated in the gut by MAO, and patients taking MAOIs must be warned about the dangers of eating tyramine-rich foods.

268. The answer is a. (*Katzung, p 499.*) Of the listed antidepressants, only amitriptyline, a tricyclic, causes adverse effects related to blockade of muscarinic acetylcholine receptors. Both trazodone and amitriptyline cause adverse effects related to α-adrenoreceptor blockade.

269. The answer is a. (*Hardman, p 444.*) This patient has the serotonin syndrome. Serotonin is already present in increased amounts in synapses because of blockade of its reuptake by the SSRIs. The amount of serotonin that is present is further increased when breakdown by MAO is inhibited. The serotonin syndrome can be life threatening.

270. The answer is c. (*Hardman, p 408.*) Clozapine differs from other neuroleptic agents in that it can induce seizures in nonepileptic patients. In patients with a history of epileptic seizures for which they are not receiving treatment, stimulation of seizures can occur following the administration of neuroleptic agents because they lower seizure threshold and cause brain discharge patterns reminiscent of epileptic seizure disorders.

271. The answer is d. (*Katzung, p 482.*) Although many antipsychotic agents can cause orthostatic hypotension, chlorpromazine is the most likely choice of the agents above for causing this adverse effect.

272. The answer is d. (*Hardman, p 564.*) A long-acting benzodiazepine, such as diazepam, is effective in blocking the secobarbital withdrawal symptoms. The anxiolytic effects of buspirone take several days to develop, obviating its use for acute severe anxiety.

273. The answer is d. (*Hardman, p 564. Katzung, pp 370, 1013.*) Flumazenil is a competitive antagonist of benzodiazepines at the GABA receptor. Repeated administration is necessary because of its short half-life relative to that of most benzodiazepines.

274. The answer is b. *(Hardman, pp 365–367.)* Benzodiazepines, such as diazepam, bind to the GABA receptor/ion channel complex, enhancing GABA-induced Cl^- currents related to more frequent bursts of Cl^- channel opening by GABA.

275. The answer is d. *(Katzung, pp 411, 1029.)* An increased incidence of spina bifida may occur with the use of valproic acid during pregnancy. Cardiovascular, orofacial, and digital abnormalities may also occur. The main issue with the use of phenobarbital or primidone (metabolite is phenobarbital) for the fetus is neonatal dependence on barbiturates.

276. The answer is c. *(Hardman, p 340. Katzung, p 437.)* Of the listed agents, only bupivacaine is an amide. Allergy to amide-type local anesthetics is much less frequent than with ester-type local anesthetics, such as benzocaine; patients who demonstrate an allergy to one such drug will be allergic to all of them.

277. The answer is a. *(Hardman, p 338. Katzung, pp 438–439.)* Ester-type local anesthetics are mainly hydrolyzed by pseudocholinesterases. Amide-type local anesthetics are hydrolyzed by microsomal enzymes in the liver. Of the listed agents, only lidocaine is an amide and can be influenced by liver dysfunction.

278. The answer is a. *(Hardman, p 906. Katzung, p 1127.)* Cimetidine inhibits the activity of cytochrome P450, slowing benzodiazepam metabolism.

279. The answer is b. *(Hardman, p 448. Katzung, pp 493, 1130.)* Some NSAIDs can increase proximal tubular reabsorption of lithium salts, which can create toxic levels of lithium in the plasma.

Autonomic Nervous System

Questions

DIRECTIONS: Each item below contains a question or incomplete statement followed by suggested responses. Select the **one best** response to each question.

280. Of the many types of adrenergic receptors found throughout the body, which is most likely responsible for the cardiac stimulation that is observed following an intravenous injection of epinephrine?

a. α_1-adrenergic receptors
b. α_2-adrenergic receptors
c. β_1-adrenergic receptors
d. β_2-adrenergic receptors
e. β_3-adrenergic receptors

281. The enzyme that is inhibited by echothiophate iodide is

a. Tyrosine hydroxylase
b. Acetylcholinesterase (AChE)
c. Catechol-O-methyltransferase (COMT)
d. Monoamine oxidase (MAO)
e. Carbonic anhydrase

282. Applied to the skin in a transdermal patch (transdermal therapeutic delivery system), this drug is used to prevent or reduce the occurrence of nausea and vomiting that are associated with motion sickness.

a. Diphenhydramine
b. Chlorpromazine
c. Ondansetron
d. Dimenhydrinate
e. Scopolamine

283. The nonselective β-adrenergic blocking agent that is also a competitive antagonist at α_1-adrenoceptors is

a. Timolol
b. Nadolol
c. Pindolol
d. Acebutolol
e. Labetalol

284. The contractile effect of various doses of norepinephrine (NE) (X) alone on vascular smooth muscle is represented in the figure below.

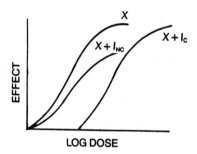

When combined with an antagonist (I_C or I_{NC}), a shift in the dose-response curve occurs. The curve labeled $X + I_{NC}$ would most likely occur when vascular smooth muscle is treated with NE in the presence of

a. Terazosin
b. Phentolamine
c. Labetalol
d. Phenoxybenzamine
e. Prazosin

285. The reversible cholinesterase inhibitor indicated in the treatment of Alzheimer's disease is

a. Tacrine
b. Edrophonium
c. Neostigmine
d. Pyridostigmine
e. Ambenonium

286. Hypotension, bradycardia, respiratory depression, and muscle weakness, all unresponsive to atropine and neostigmine, would most likely be due to

a. Diazoxide
b. Isofluorphate
c. Tubocurarine
d. Nicotine
e. Pilocarpine

287. Ritodrine hydrochloride is used in the treatment of

a. Parkinson's disease
b. Bronchial asthma
c. Depression
d. Hypertension
e. Premature labor

288. The skeletal muscle relaxant that acts directly on the contractile mechanism of the muscle fibers is

a. Gallamine
b. Baclofen
c. Pancuronium
d. Cyclobenzaprine
e. Dantrolene

289. A predictably dangerous side effect of nadolol that constitutes a contraindication to its clinical use in susceptible patients is the induction of

a. Hypertension
b. Cardiac arrhythmia
c. Asthmatic attacks
d. Respiratory depression
e. Hypersensitivity

290. All of the following drugs are used topically in the treatment of chronic wide-angle glaucoma. Which of these agents reduces intraocular pressure by decreasing the formation of the aqueous humor?

a. Timolol
b. Echothiophate
c. Pilocarpine
d. Isofluorphate
e. Physostigmine

291. The cholinomimetic drug that is useful for treating postoperative abdominal distention and gastric atony is

a. Acetylcholine (ACh)
b. Methacholine
c. Carbachol
d. Bethanechol
e. Pilocarpine

292. Neostigmine will effectively antagonize skeletal muscle relaxation produced by

a. Pancuronium
b. Succinylcholine
c. Diazepam
d. Baclofen
e. Nicotine

293. Pralidoxime chloride is a drug that

a. Reduces the vesicular stores of catecholamines in adrenergic and dopaminergic neurons
b. Blocks the active transport of choline into cholinergic neurons
c. Reactivates cholinesterases that have been inhibited by organophosphate cholinesterase inhibitors
d. Stimulates the activity of phospholipase C with increased formation of inositol triphosphate
e. Inhibits the reuptake of biogenic amines into nerve terminals

294. Which of the following antimuscarinic drugs is used by inhalation in the treatment of bronchial asthma?

a. Dicyclomine hydrochloride
b. Cyclopentolate hydrochloride
c. Ipratropium bromide
d. Methscopolamine bromide
e. Trihexyphenidyl hydrochloride

295. The cholinesterase inhibitor that is used in the diagnosis of myasthenia gravis is

a. Edrophonium chloride
b. Ambenonium chloride
c. Malathion
d. Physostigmine salicylate
e. Pyridostigmine bromide

296. Epinephrine may be mixed with certain anesthetics, such as procaine, in order to

a. Stimulate local wound repair
b. Promote hemostasis
c. Enhance their interaction with neural membranes and their ability to depress nerve conduction
d. Retard their systemic absorption
e. Facilitate their distribution along nerves and fascial planes

297. The skeletal muscles that are most sensitive to the action of tubocurarine are the

a. Muscles of the trunk
b. Muscles of the arms and legs
c. Respiratory muscles
d. Muscles of the head, neck, and face
e. Abdominal muscles

298. The drug of choice for the treatment of anaphylactic shock is

a. Epinephrine
b. NE
c. Isoproterenol
d. Diphenhydramine
e. Atropine

299. Both phentolamine and prazosin

a. Are competitive antagonists at α_1-adrenergic receptors
b. Have potent direct vasodilator actions on vascular smooth muscle
c. Enhance gastric acid secretion through a histamine-like effect
d. Cause hypotension and bradycardia
e. Are used chronically for the treatment of primary hypotension

300. A 60-year-old male with congestive heart failure (CHF) is treated with dobutamine. Select the mechanism of action of dobutamine.

a. α-adrenergic agonist
b. α-adrenergic antagonist
c. β-adrenergic agonist
d. β-adrenergic antagonist
e. Mixed α and β agonist
f. Mixed α and β antagonist

301. A 58-year-old male with angina is treated with atenolol. Select the mechanism of action of atenolol.

a. α-adrenergic agonist
b. α-adrenergic antagonist
c. β-adrenergic agonist
d. β-adrenergic antagonist
e. Mixed α and β agonist
f. Mixed α and β antagonist

302. A 75-year-old female with CHF is treated with carvedilol. Select the mechanism of action of carvedilol.

a. α-adrenergic agonist
b. α-adrenergic antagonist
c. β-adrenergic agonist
d. β-adrenergic antagonist
e. Mixed α and β agonist
f. Mixed α and β antagonist

303. A 35-year-old male with a pheochromocytoma is treated with labetalol. Select the mechanism of action of labetalol.

a. α-adrenergic agonist
b. α-adrenergic antagonist
c. β-adrenergic agonist
d. β-adrenergic antagonist
e. Mixed α and β agonist
f. Mixed α and β antagonist

304. Which of the following agents will increase pulse pressure?

a. Metoprolol
b. Dopamine
c. Isoproterenol
d. Epinephrine
e. Albuterol

305. A male patient is brought to the emergency department (ED) following ingestion of an unknown substance. He is found to have an elevated temperature, hot and flushed skin, dilated pupils, and tachycardia. Of the following, which would most likely cause these findings?

a. Propranolol
b. Methylphenidate
c. Prazosin
d. Guanethidine
e. Atropine

306. Of the following structures, which does not respond to β-adrenergic receptor stimulation?

a. Ciliary muscle of the iris
b. Radial muscle of the iris
c. Bronchial muscle
d. Atrioventricular (AV) node
e. Sinoatrial (SA) node

307. A 16-year-old male treated for bronchial asthma develops skeletal muscle tremors. Which of the following agents may be responsible for this finding?

a. Ipratropium
b. Zileuton
c. Beclomethasone
d. Cromolyn
e. Salmeterol

308. Of the following, which will not be blocked by atropine and scopolamine?

a. Bradycardia
b. Salivary secretion
c. Bronchoconstriction
d. Skeletal muscle contraction
e. Miosis

309. Which of the following agents should a patient take for a stuffy, runny nose?

a. Oxymetazoline
b. Albuterol
c. Clonidine
d. Terbutaline
e. Metoprolol

310. A 65-year-old male has a blood pressure of 170/105 mmHg. Which of the following would be effective in lowering this patient's blood pressure?

a. Methylphenidate
b. Terbutaline
c. Dobutamine
d. Pancuronium
e. Prazosin
f. Scopalamine

311. A 10-year-old male displays hyperactivity and is unable to focus on his schoolwork because of an inability to focus on the activity. Which of the following might prove effective in this patient?

a. Methylphenidate
b. Terbutaline
c. Dobutamine
d. Pancuronium
e. Prazosin
f. Scopalamine

312. Nicotine in low doses may cause

a. Decreased tone and motor activity of the small intestine
b. Stimulation of the respiratory rate and depth
c. Miosis
d. Bradycardia

313. Which of the following agents might mask the hypoglycemia in treated diabetics?

a. An α-adrenergic agonist
b. An α-adrenergic antagonist
c. A β-adrenergic agonist
d. A β-adrenergic antagonist
e. A cholinergic agonist
f. A cholinergic antagonist

314. Of the following effects, which is not elicited by activation of the parasympathetic nervous system?

a. Decreased heart rate
b. Increased tone of longitudinal smooth muscles of the intestine
c. Contraction of skeletal muscles
d. Contraction of the detrusor of the urinary bladder
e. Secretion of fluid from the lacrimal glands

315. Which of the following occurs in the treatment of glaucoma with a β-adrenergic antagonist?

a. Decreased aqueous humor secretion
b. Pupillary dilator muscle fiber contraction
c. Dilation of the uveoscleral veins
d. Direct opening of the trabecular meshwork
e. Circular pupillary constrictor muscle contraction

DIRECTIONS: Each group of questions below consists of lettered options followed by a set of numbered items. For each numbered item, select the **one** lettered option with which it is **most** closely associated. Each lettered option may be used once, more than once, or not at all.

Questions 316–317

For each patient, which drug was given?

a. Diazepam
b. Doxazosin
c. Scopolamine
d. Cyclobenzaprine
e. Propantheline
f. Atracurium
g. Atenolol
h. Baclofen
i. Timolol
j. Phentolamine

316. A 65-year-old male complains of losing his vision. Retinal examination reveals optic nerve cupping. Peripheral vision loss is observed on visual field tests, and his intraocular pressure is increased. Following treatment with a drug, he has improved visual acuity and decreased intraocular pressure.

317. A 30-year-old female is being prepared for anesthesia before exploratory surgery for a mass in her neck. In addition to using an inhalation anesthetic, a drug is given that causes complete paralysis of the skeletal muscles.

Questions 318–320

For each anatomic site listed, select the catecholamine neurotransmitter found in the highest amounts.

a. Dopamine
b. 5-hydroxytryptamine (5-HT)
c. Epinephrine
d. NE
e. ACh

318. Adrenergic fibers

319. Adrenal medulla

320. Caudate nucleus

Questions 321–323

The figure below illustrates proposed sites of action of drugs. For each drug listed, select the site of action that the drug is most likely to inhibit (α, α receptor; β, β receptor; COMT, catechol-O-methyltransferase; MAO, monoamine oxidase; NE, norepinephrine; NMN, normetanephrine).

a. α receptor
b. β receptor
c.
d.
e.
f.
g.
h.
i.
j.

SYMPATHETIC NEUROEFFECTOR JUNCTION

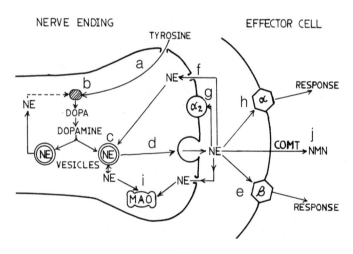

321. Reserpine

322. Esmolol

323. Tranylcypromine

Questions 324–326

For each patient, select the mechanism of action that is most likely associated with the administered drug.

a. α-adrenergic antagonist
b. β-adrenergic antagonist
c. Calcium (Ca) channel antagonist
d. Carbonic anhydrase inhibitor
e. Histamine (H_1) receptor antagonist
f. H_2 receptor antagonist
g. MAOI
h. Sodium/potassium/(Na^+,K^+) adenosine triphosphatase (ATPase) inhibitor
i. Na^+ channel antagonist
j. Serotonin receptor antagonist

324. A 16-year-old female has a two-year history of runny nose and itchy eyes from mid-August through mid-October. Chlorpheniramine is given and provides symptomatic relief.

325. A 66-year-old male with a one-year history of essential hypertension has minimal response to diet and a diuretic. His blood pressure is now 160/105 mmHg. The diuretic is discontinued, and propranolol is given.

326. During the past year, a 38-year-old female has become progressively depressed and now refuses to leave her house. Physical examination and blood chemistries are negative. She is given phenelzine, which diminishes her depression and enables her to leave her house.

Questions 327–329

For each of the neurotransmitters below, select the amino acid from which it is synthesized.

a. Tyrosine
b. Serine
c. Histidine
d. Tryptophan
e. Hydroxyproline

327. Epinephrine

328. Histamine

329. Serotonin

Questions 330–332

Match the descriptions of use with the appropriate drug.
a. Pilocarpine
b. Methylphenidate
c. Propranolol
d. Ritodrine
e. Phenoxybenzamine

330. Used in pheochromocytoma

331. Used in thyroid storm

332. Used in glaucoma

Questions 333–335

For each of the drugs listed below, select its appropriate site of action in the ACh system that is diagrammed.

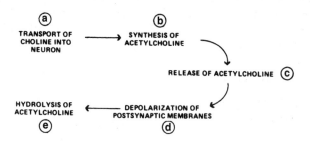

333. Botulinus toxin

334. Hemicholinium

335. Muscarine in poisonous mushrooms

Autonomic Nervous System

Answers

280. The answer is c. *(Hardman, pp 205–208.)* Stimulation of both the contractile and rhythmic effects of epinephrine on the heart is mediated through activation of postsynaptic β_1-adrenergic receptors. These receptor sites mediate an epinephrine-induced increased firing rate of the SA node, increased conduction velocity through the AV node and the His-Purkinje system, and increased contractility and conduction velocity of atrial and ventricular muscle. Epinephrine activation of α adrenoceptors does not affect cardiac function. β_2-adrenergic receptors play a minor role in cardiac stimulation. They are more important in the relaxation of tracheobronchial smooth muscle, relaxation of the detrusor of the urinary bladder, dilation of arterioles that serve skeletal muscles, and increased secretion of insulin by the pancreas. Lipolysis in fat cells and melatonin secretion by the pineal gland appear to involve stimulation of β_3-adrenergic receptors.

281. The answer is b. *(Hardman, pp 166–167.)* Echothiophate iodide is a long-acting (irreversible) cholinesterase inhibitor. It is used topically in the eye for the treatment of various types of glaucoma. Maximum reduction of intraocular pressure occurs within 24 h, and the effect may persist for several days. The drug is a water-soluble compound, which affords it a practical advantage over the lipid-soluble isofluorphate (another cholinesterase inhibitor used to treat glaucoma).

282. The answer is e. *(Hardman, p 930.)* All the drugs listed in the question are used as antiemetics. Chlorpromazine is a general antiemetic, used orally, rectally, or by injection for the control of nausea and vomiting that is caused by conditions that are not necessarily defined. Ondansetron is indicated in the oral or intravenous route for the prevention of nausea and vomiting caused by cancer chemotherapy. Diphenhydramine and dimenhydrinate are used orally for the active and prophylactic treatment of motion sickness. Scopolamine is a transdermal preparation used in the prevention of motion sickness. The drug is incorporated into a bandage-like adhesive unit that is placed behind the ear. The scopolamine delivered in this manner is well absorbed and maintains an effect for up to 72 h. Other drugs that are prepared for transdermal delivery include clonidine (an antihypertensive agent), estradiol (an estrogen), fentanyl (an opioid analgesic), nicotine (a smoking deterrent), nitroglycerin (an antianginal drug), and testosterone (an androgen).

283. The answer is e. *(Hardman, pp 235–239.)* With the exception of acebutolol—which is classified as a *cardioselective,* or selective, β_1-adrenergic blocking agent—all of the drugs listed are considered to be nonselective β-adrenergic blocking agents because they will competitively antagonize agonists at both β_1- and β_2-adrenergic receptor sites. Labetalol is unique in that it is, at therapeutic doses, also a competitive antagonist at α_1-adrenergic receptors. The drug has more potent blocking activity at β-adrenoceptors; the potency ratio for α:β blockade is 1:3 for the oral route and 1:7 after intravenous administration. Similar to the other β-adrenergic blocking drugs, labetalol is indicated for the treatment of essential hypertension; however, because of the α_1-adrenergic blocking activity, blood pressure is often decreased more in the standing than in the supine position, and symptoms of postural hypotension can occur.

284. The answer is d. *(Katzung, pp 28–30.)* Competitive antagonists produce a parallel shift to the right in the dose-response curve of an agonist without a reduction in the maximal effect. This type of inhibition of agonist response is due to the reversible binding of the antagonist with the affected receptor site(s); this is exemplified in the curve shown for the agonist NE (X) plus an antagonist (I_{NC}). Noncompetitive antagonists prevent an agonist from inducing any effect at a given receptor site and thus reduce the number of receptor sites that can be stimulated by an agonist. These compounds produce a nonparallel shift in the dose-response curve of the agonist and a diminution in the maximum response, as shown by the curve labeled $X + I_{NC}$. Norepinephrine (NE) contracts vascular smooth muscle by binding to and activating α_1-adrenergic receptors. Phentolamine, prazosin, terazosin, and labetalol all bind to α_1-adrenergic receptors, but fail to activate them. Because the action of these compounds is reversible, these drugs act as competitive antagonists of NE at these receptor sites. Phenoxybenzamine is an alkylating agent that forms a stable covalent bond with both α_1- and α_2-adrenergic receptors. This long-lasting receptor blockade cannot be overcome by competition with an agonist. Therefore, in contrast to the other drugs listed, blockade with phenoxybenzamine is not reversible, is referred to as nonequilibrium receptor blockade, and in the presence of an α-adrenergic receptor agonist such as NE will result in a dose-response curve exemplified by curve $X + I_{NC}$.

285. The answer is a. *(Katzung, p 1040.)* Patients with Alzheimer's disease present with progressive impairment of memory and cognitive functions such as a lack of attention, disturbed language function, and an inability to complete common tasks. Although the exact defect in the central nervous system (CNS) has not been elucidated, evidence suggests that a reduction in cholinergic nerve function is largely responsible for the symptoms.

Tacrine has been found to be somewhat effective in patients with mild-to-moderate symptoms of this disease for improvement of cognitive functions. The drug is primarily a reversible cholinesterase inhibitor that increases the concentration of functional ACh in the brain. However, the pharmacology of tacrine is complex; the drug also acts as a muscarinic receptor modulator in that it has partial agonistic activity, as well as weak antagonistic activity on muscarinic receptors in the CNS. In addition, tacrine appears to enhance the release of ACh from cholinergic nerves, and it may alter the concentrations of other neurotransmitters such as dopamine and NE.

Of all of the reversible cholinesterase inhibitors, only tacrine and physostigmine cross the blood-brain barrier in sufficient amounts to make these compounds useful for disorders involving the CNS. Physostigmine has been tried as a therapy for Alzheimer's disease; however, it is more commonly used to antagonize the effects of toxic concentrations of drugs with antimuscarinic properties, including atropine, antihistamines, phenothiazines, and tricyclic antidepressants. Neostigmine, pyridostigmine, and ambenonium are used mainly in the treatment of myasthenia gravis; edrophonium is useful for the diagnosis of this muscular disease.

286. The answer is d. *(Hardman, pp 192–193.)* Nicotine is a depolarizing ganglionic blocking agent that initially stimulates and then blocks nicotinic muscular (NM) (skeletal muscle) and nicotinic neural (NN) (parasympathetic ganglia) cholinergic receptors. Blockade of the sympathetic division of the autonomic nervous system (ANS) results in arteriolar vasodilation, bradycardia, and hypotension. Blockade at the neuromuscular junction leads to muscle weakness and respiratory depression caused by interference with the function of the diaphragm and intercostal muscles. Atropine, a muscarinic receptor blocker, would be an effective antagonist, as would neostigmine, a cholinesterase inhibitor. Pilocarpine and isofluorphate are cholinomimetics and can be antagonized by atropine; the effects of tubocurarine can be inhibited by neostigmine. Diazoxide, a vasodilator, would cause tachycardia, rather than bradycardia.

287. The answer is e. (*Hardman, p 215.*) Ritodrine hydrochloride is a selective β_2-adrenergic agonist that relaxes uterine smooth muscle. It also has the other effects attributable to β-adrenergic receptor stimulants, such as bronchodilation, cardiac stimulation, enhanced renin secretion, and hyperglycemia.

288. The answer is e. (*Katzung, pp 459–460.*) There are three major classes of skeletal muscle relaxants: (1) peripherally acting, (2) centrally acting, and (3) direct-acting. The peripherally acting drugs include the nondepolarizing (e.g., tubocurarine, gallamine, pancuronium) and depolarizing (e.g., succinylcholine, decamethonium) neuromuscular blockers that antagonize ACh at the muscle endplate (i.e., at NM receptors). Centrally acting skeletal muscle relaxants (e.g., diazepam, cyclobenzaprine, baclofen) interfere with transmission along the monosynaptic and polysynaptic neural pathways in the spinal cord. Dantrolene, the only direct-acting skeletal muscle relaxant, affects the excitation-contraction coupling mechanism of skeletal muscle by depressing the release of ionic Ca from the sarcoplasmic reticulum to the myoplasma. The drug is also useful in the prevention and management of malignant hyperthermia induced by general anesthetics.

289. The answer is c. (*Hardman, pp 233–235.*) The chief danger of therapy with β-adrenergic blocking agents, such as nadolol and propranolol, is associated with the blockade itself. β-adrenergic blockade results in an increase in airway resistance that can be fatal in asthmatic patients. Hypersensitivity reactions such as rash, fever, and purpura are rare and necessitate discontinuation of therapy.

290. The answer is a. (*Hardman, pp 146–147, 167.*) When applied topically to the eye, both the direct-acting cholinomimetic agents (e.g., pilocarpine) and those cholinomimetic drugs that act by inhibition of AChE (e.g., echothiophate, isofluorphate, and physostigmine) cause miosis by contracting the sphincter muscle of the iris and reducing ocular pressure by contracting the ciliary muscle. In patients with glaucoma, this latter effect permits greater drainage of the aqueous humor through the trabecular meshwork in the canal of Schlemm and a reduction in resistance to outflow of the aqueous humor. Certain β-adrenergic blocking agents (e.g., timolol and levobunolol) applied to the eye are also very useful in treating chronic wide-angle glaucoma. These drugs appear to act by decreasing the secretion (or formation) of the aqueous humor by antagonizing the effect of circulating catecholamines on β-adrenergic receptors in the ciliary epithelium.

291. The answer is d. *(Hardman, pp 143–145.)* Of the four choline esters (ACh, methacholine, carbachol, and bethanechol), the latter two drugs have the greatest agonistic activity on muscarinic receptors of the GI tract and urinary bladder. Bethanechol is used orally or by subcutaneous injection as a stimulant of the smooth muscles of the GI tract (for cases of postoperative abdominal distention, gastric atony, and retention or gastroparesis) and the urinary bladder (for nonobstructive postoperative and postpartum urinary retention). Carbachol is not used for these purposes due to significant activity at nicotinic receptors at autonomic ganglia; the drug is useful as a miotic for treating glaucoma and in certain types of ocular surgery. Acetylcholine is occasionally used topically during cataract surgery; metacholine is used by inhalation for the diagnosis of bronchial hyperreactivity in patients who do not have clinically apparent asthma. Pilocarpine (a naturally occurring alkaloid) is a drug of choice for the treatment of glaucoma.

292. The answer is a. *(Hardman, pp 162–165.)* Anticholinesterase agents, such as neostigmine, will delay the catabolism of ACh that is released from parasympathetic autonomic and somatic nerve terminals. At the neuromuscular junction, this results in increased competition for the NM receptors by ACh (the agonist) and the curariform drugs (the antagonists) such as tubocurarine and pancuronium. In addition, neostigmine has a direct stimulating action on the skeletal muscle junction, which enhances its ability to antagonize the competitive neuromuscular blockers. The activity of succinylcholine at the neuromuscular junction will be exacerbated by neostigmine, because succinylcholine is inactivated by AChE. The skeletal muscle relaxation that may result from toxic doses of nicotine-blocking NM receptors will be unaffected by neostigmine. Diazepam and baclofen are centrally acting skeletal muscle relaxants whose effects are not altered by the peripheral actions of neostigmine.

293. The answer is c. (*Hardman, pp 170–171.*) Organophosphate cholinesterase inhibitors react with both AChE and serum cholinesterase (pseudocholinesterase) by phosphorylating the enzymes, thus rendering them inactive, inasmuch as the phosphorylated enzyme hydrolyzes esters very slowly. Pralidoxime chloride (2-PAM Cl⁻) is an oxime derivative that can cause dephosphorylation of the enzyme if it is administered within a short time after the organophosphate. If it is not administered promptly, the phosphorylated enzyme will lose an alkyl or alkoxy group (a process called *aging*), leaving a more stable phosphorylated enzyme that then cannot be dephosphorylated. The time period during which this occurs depends upon the nature of the phosphoryl group and the rapidity with which the organophosphate compound affects the enzyme. This can be from a few seconds to several hours.

294. The answer is c. (*Hardman, pp 156–158.*) A wide variety of clinical conditions are treated with antimuscarinic drugs. Dicyclomine hydrochloride and methscopolamine bromide are used to reduce GI motility, although side effects—dryness of the mouth, loss of visual accommodation, and difficulty in urination—may limit their acceptance by patients. Cyclopentolate hydrochloride is used in ophthalmology for its mydriatic and cycloplegic properties during refraction of the eye. Trihexyphenidyl hydrochloride is one of the important antimuscarinic compounds used in the treatment of parkinsonism. For bronchodilation in patients with bronchial asthma and other bronchospastic diseases, ipratropium bromide is used by inhalation. Systemic adverse reactions are low because the actions are largely confined to the mouth and airways.

295. The answer is a. (*Hardman, pp 161–169.*) Although all of the listed compounds inhibit the activity of the cholinesterases, only edrophonium chloride is used in the diagnosis of myasthenia gravis. The drug has a more rapid onset of action (1 to 3 min following intravenous administration) and a shorter duration of action (approximately 5 to 10 min) than pyridostigmine bromide. It is more water-soluble than physostigmine salicylate and, therefore, produces no clinically significant adverse effects on the CNS. Pyridostigmine bromide is used in the treatment of this muscle weakness disease. Physostigmine salicylate is indicated topically for the treatment of glaucomas and is also a valuable drug for treating toxicity of anticholinergic drugs such as atropine. Malathion is an anticholinesterase that is used topically for the treatment of head lice and is never used internally.

296. The answer is d. (*Hardman, p 336.*) The addition of a vasoconstrictor, such as epinephrine or phenylephrine, to certain short-acting, local anesthetics is a common practice in order to prevent the rapid systemic absorption of the local anesthetics, to prolong the local action, and to decrease the potential systemic reactions. Some local anesthetics cause vasodilation, which allows more compound to escape the tissue and enter the blood. Procaine is an ester-type local anesthetic with a short duration of action due to rather rapid biotransformation in the plasma by cholinesterases. The duration of action of the drug during infiltration anesthesia is greatly increased by the addition of epinephrine, which reduces the vasodilation caused by procaine.

297. The answer is d. (*Hardman, pp 183–185.*) Flaccid paralysis of all skeletal muscles can be produced by the intravenous administration of large doses of a neuromuscular blocking agent, such as tubocurarine. However, not all skeletal musculature is equally sensitive to the action of these drugs. The muscles that produce fine movements (e.g., the extraocular muscles, fingers, and muscles of the head, face, and neck) are most sensitive to these drugs. Muscles of the trunk, abdomen, and extremities are relaxed next, and the respiratory muscles (i.e., the intercostals and the diaphragm) are the most resistant to the action of tubocurarine.

298. The answer is a. (*Hardman, p 224.*) Epinephrine is the drug of choice to relieve the symptoms of an acute, systemic, immediate hypersensitivity reaction to an allergen (anaphylactic shock). Subcutaneous administration of a 1:1000 solution of epinephrine rapidly relieves itching and urticaria, and this may save the life of the patient when laryngeal edema and bronchospasm threaten suffocation and severe hypotension and cardiac arrhythmias become life-endangering. Norepinephrine, isoproterenol, and atropine are ineffective therapies. Angioedema is responsive to antihistamines (e.g., diphenhydramine), but epinephrine is necessary in the event of a severe reaction.

299. The answer is a. *(Hardman, pp 228–229.)* Phentolamine is a non-selective α-adrenergic receptor blocker (i.e., it has affinity for both α$_1$- and α$_2$-adrenergic receptor sites). It also has a prominent direct relaxant (musculotropic spasmolytic) effect on arterioles, which results in vasodilation and reflex tachycardia. In addition, phentolamine can block the effects of serotonin and will increase hydrochloric acid and pepsin secretion from the stomach. Phentolamine is used for the short-term control of hypertension in patients with pheochromocytoma (i.e., a type of secondary hypertension); because of the high incidence of tachycardia associated with the compound, it is not used chronically for the treatment of essential hypertension.

Prazosin is a selective α$_1$-adrenergic receptor antagonist that, at therapeutic doses, has little activity at α$_2$-adrenergic receptors and clinically insignificant direct vasodilating activity. The drug does not cause the other effects attributed to phentolamine. Most important, it produces less tachycardia than does phentolamine and, therefore, is useful in the treatment of essential hypertension.

300. The answer is e. *(Katzung, pp 130–131, 209.)* Dobutamine is a β$_1$-selective agonist with α$_1$-selective activity. The racemic mixture contains the (+) isomer, which is predominantly a potent β$_1$ agonist with some α$_1$ antagonist effects, while the (−) isomer is a potent α$_1$ agonist. Functionally, these properties of the isomers make dobutamine a mixed α and β agonist. Dobutamine is used clinically as a β$_1$-selective agonist. It is useful in CHF because of its ability to increase cardiac output while causing a decrease in ventricular filling pressure. It may not benefit patients with ischemic heart disease because it tends to increase heart rate and myocardial oxygen demand.

301. The answer is d. *(Katzung, pp 147–148, 195.)* Atenolol is a β$_1$-specific antagonist. It is effective in decreasing symptoms of angina. The benefits that are gained from beta-blocking agents are decreased heart rate, blood pressure, and myocardial contractility, leading to a decrease in myocardial oxygen demand.

302. The answer is f. *(Katzung, pp 167, 213.)* Carvedilol is a racemic mixture, with the S(−) isomer being a nonselective β-adrenergic antagonist and both its S(−) and R(+) isomers being an α-adrenergic antagonist. Carvedilol and β-adrenergic antagonists are known to increase survival in CHF.

303. The answer is f. *(Katzung, p 167. Hardman, pp 237–238.)* Labetalol has potent α and β antagonist actions, due to the specific components of its racemic mixture of four isomeric compounds. Cardiac output and heart rate change minimally, while blood pressure decreases due to a overall reduction in peripheral resistance. The combined α and β antagonism has been found to be of advantage in treating pheochromocytomas.

304. The answer is d. *(Katzung, p 130.)* Epinephrine has a positive ionotropic and chronotropic effect on the heart because of its β_1-adrenergic activity. It also has α-adrenergic activity that causes vasoconstriction in the vascular beds. These actions result in a rise in systolic blood pressure. Epinephrine also has β_2-adrenergic activity, which causes vasodilation in skeletal muscle. Because of this latter effect, total peripheral resistance can fall, resulting in a drop in diastolic pressure, particularly at low doses of epinephrine.

305. The answer is e. *(Katzung, p 116).* High concentrations of atropine block all parasympathetic function. The patient usually presents with an array of symptoms and signs that include dry mouth, dilated pupils, tachycardia, red and hot skin, and delirium. Hyperthermia may occur, particularly in very young children.

306. The answer is b. *(Katzung, pp 85, 90.)* The radial muscle of the iris contains predominantly α-adrenergic receptors; when exposed to such α-receptor agonists as phenylephrine, the muscle contracts, resulting in mydriasis. Miosis occurs when the ciliary muscle, which contains β receptors, relaxes. Bronchial muscle, the AV node, and the SA node are among other sites that contain β receptors and respond to β-adrenergic agonists.

307. The answer is e. *(Katzung, pp 340–342.)* Salmeterol is a long-acting β_2-adrenergic agonist that is effective in asthma prophylaxis. Skeletal muscle tremor is associated with β_2-adrenergic agonists, whether short acting or not. Other shorter-acting β_2-adrenergic agonists include albuterol and terbutaline.

308. The answer is d. *(Hardman, pp 142–143.)* ACh will stimulate both muscarinic and nicotinic receptors. Skeletal muscle contraction is mediated through NM receptors, and ganglionic stimulation is an effect of NN receptors. All of the other effects listed in the question occur following muscarinic receptor activation and will be blocked by atropine and scopolamine, both of which are muscarinic receptor antagonists. Skeletal muscle contraction will not be affected by these drugs; rather, a neuromuscular blocker (e.g., tubocurarine) is required to antagonize this effect of ACh.

309. The answer is a. *(Katzung, p 130.)* Oxymetazoline is an α-adrenergic agonist. It causes vasoconstriction of the nasal mucosa. Because of its long duration of action, it is useful in decreasing nasal congestion, especially due to upper respiratory infections. Pseudoephedrine and phenylephrine are other α-adrenergic agonists used for similar purposes.

310. The answer is e. *(Katzung, pp 141, 168.)* Prazosin blocks α_1-adrenergic receptors in arterioles, thereby decreasing peripheral resistance and leading to a decrease in blood pressure. Orthostatic hypotension can occur, particularly after a first dose.

311. The answer is a. *(Hardman, p 221. Katzung, p 131.)* Methylphenidate is similar to amphetamine and acts as a CNS stimulant, with more pronounced effects on mental than on motor activities. It is effective in the treatment of narcolepsy and attention-deficit hyperactivity disorders.

312. The answer is b. *(Hardman, pp 192–193.)* Nicotine is a depolarizing ganglionic blocking agent; that is, it stimulates nicotinic receptors in low doses and predominantly blocks at high-dose levels. The effect of nicotine on a particular tissue or organ depends on the relative contribution to the function made by each division of the ANS. The effects on the cardiovascular system are complex. Stimulation of the cardiac vagal ganglia causes bradycardia. This is countered by sympathetic stimulation to the heart (tachycardia), blood vessels (vasoconstriction), and adrenal medulla (catecholamine release: tachycardia and vasoconstriction). Thus, the net effect of nicotine on the heart is tachycardia, not bradycardia. Low doses of nicotine augment respiration by excitation of the chemoreceptors of the carotid body and aortic arch. Higher doses also stimulate the medullary respiratory center and increase respiration through CNS activity. Large amounts of nicotine cause respiratory failure from medullary paralysis and blockade of the skeletal muscles of respiration.

313. The answer is d. *(Hardman, pp 235–237. Katzung, pp 151–152.)* β-adrenergic antagonists should be used with caution in diabetic patients who are prone to hypoglycemia because β-adrenergic antagonists may mask the warning signs of acute hypoglycemia (e.g., tachycardia). They most likely do this by blocking glycogenolysis and the mobilization of glucose in response to hypoglycemia that is stimulated by catecholamines.

314. The answer is c. *(Hardman, pp 115–117.)* Cholinergic impulses arising from the parasympathetic division of the ANS affect many tissues and organs throughout the body. Physiologically, this system is concerned primarily with the functions of energy conservation and maintenance of organ function during periods of reduced activity. Slowed heart rate, reduced blood pressure, increased GI motility, emptying of the urinary bladder, and stimulation of secretions from the pancreas, salivary glands, lacrimal glands, and bronchial and nasopharyngeal glands are all effects observed that are due to activation of this nervous system. However, skeletal muscle contraction is mediated through activation of the somatic nervous system, not the ANS.

315. The answer is a. *(Katzung, p 88.)* The secretion of aqueous humor is effected by β-adrenergic receptors located on ciliary epithelia. The use of β-adrenergic antagonists decreases secretory activity and lowers intraocular pressure. Muscarinic agents induce contraction in the circular pupillary constrictor muscles. Ciliary muscle contraction facilitates pore opening of the trabecular meshwork leading to outflow of the aqueous humor. α-adrenergic agonists cause contraction of the radially oriented pupillary dilator muscles.

316. The answer is i. *(Hardman, p 237.)* Timolol is a β-adrenergic receptor antagonist that does not show selectivity for β_1 or β_2 adrenoceptors;

therefore, it decreases heart rate by blocking the action of endogenous catecholamines. Timolol, used to lower intraocular pressure in patients with chronic open-angle glaucoma (presumably by decreasing the production of aqueous humor), is more effective than many other types of drugs for this use.

317. The answer is f. (*Hardman, p 180.*) Atracurium is a nondepolarizing neuromuscular blocking agent. Similar to tubocurarine, atracurium is a competitive antagonist of ACh at the NM receptors at the myoneural junction of skeletal muscle. At therapeutic doses, these drugs can induce complete paralysis of skeletal muscles, unlike the weaker, centrally acting skeletal muscle relaxants (e.g., diazepam, baclofen, cyclobenzaprine), which reduce spasms but do not completely block contractions. The primary therapeutic use of atracurium and other curariform drugs is as an adjunct in surgical anesthesia to relax the skeletal musculature and facilitate surgical manipulation.

318–320. The answers are 318-d, 319-c, 320-a. (*Hardman, pp 120–122.*) Norepinephrine is synthesized from dopamine by dopamine-β-oxidase, which hydroxylates the β-carbon. This enzyme is localized in the amine storage granules. Norepinephrine is found in adrenergic fibers, the adrenal medulla, and in neurons in the locus ceruleus and lateral ventral tegmental fields of the CNS.

Epinephrine is synthesized from NE in the adrenal medulla. Norepinephrine is methylated by phenylethanolamine-N-methyltransferase. Neurons containing this enzyme are also found in the CNS.

Dopamine is formed from tyrosine by hydroxylation with tyrosine hydroxylase and the removal of a CO_2 group by aromatic amino acid decarboxylase. The catecholamine is found in high concentrations in parts of the brain—the caudate nucleus, the median eminence, the tuberculum olfactorium, and the nucleus accumbens. Dopamine appears to act as an inhibitory neurotransmitter.

321–323. The answers are 321-c, 322-e, 323-i. (*Hardman, pp 238–239, 791.*) Reserpine is an adrenergic neuronal blocking agent that causes depletion of central and peripheral stores of NE and dopamine. Reserpine acts by irreversibly inhibiting the magnesium-dependent ATP transport process that functions as a carrier for biogenic amines from the cytoplasm of the neuron into the storage vesicle. Depletion of stored NE results in decreased sympathetic tone; therefore, reserpine causes vasodilation, bradycardia, and hypotension.

Esmolol hydrochloride is a competitive β-adrenergic receptor antagonist; it is selective for β_1 adrenoceptors. In contrast to pindolol, esmolol has little intrinsic sympathomimetic activity, and it differs from propranolol in that it lacks membrane stabilizing activity. Of all of the β-adrenergic blocking drugs, this compound has the shortest duration of action; because it is an ester, it is hydrolyzed rapidly by plasma esterases and must be used by the intravenous route. Esmolol is approved only for the treatment of supraventricular arrhythmias.

Tranylcypromine sulfate is an antidepressant drug and an inhibitor of MAO. Its antidepressant effect is probably due to the accumulation of NE in the brain as a consequence of inhibition of the enzyme. The other MAOI currently used as an antidepressant is phenelzine sulfate.

324. The answer is e. *(Hardman, p 587. Katzung, p 270.)* Chlorpheniramine is a competitive H_1-receptor antagonist that inhibits most responses of smooth muscle to histamine. H_1-receptor antagonists have negligible effects on H_2 or H_3 receptors.

325. The answer is b. *(Katzung, p 166.)* Propranol nonspecifically blocks β_1-adrenergic receptors. It lowers blood pressure primarily by decreasing cardiac output.

326. The answer is g. *(Hardman, pp 439–440.)* Most MAOIs are nonselective for MAO-A and -B. MAOIs mainly act on tissues regulated by sympathomimetic amines and serotonin.

327–329. The answers are 327-a, 328-c, 329-d. *(Hardman, pp 120, 250, 582–583.)* Epinephrine is made from tyrosine in a series of steps through L-dopa, dopamine, NE, and finally epinephrine. The conversion of tyrosine to dopa by tyrosine hydroxylase is the rate-limiting step in this pathway. Epinephrine constitutes about 80% of the catecholamines in the adrenal medulla. The enzyme that synthesizes epinephrine from NE is also found in certain areas of the CNS.

Histamine, formed by the decarboxylation of histidine, is stored in mast cells and basophils; some other tissues can synthesize histamine but do not store it. Histamine is released from sensitized mast cells during allergic reactions.

Serotonin is synthesized from tryptophan in two steps. Tryptophan is hydroxylated by tryptophan hydroxylase, and 5-hydroxytryptophan is decarboxylated to give serotonin. Most serotonin in the body is found in the enterochromaffin cells of the intestinal tract and the pineal gland. Platelets take up and store serotonin but do not synthesize it.

330–332. The answers are 330-e, 331-c, 332-a. *(Katzung, pp 96, 102, 142, 656.)* Propranolol, a nonselective β antagonist is effective in controlling the cardiovascular manifestations of thyroid storm. Phenoxybenzamine, an α-receptor antagonist, is used preoperatively for pheochromocytoma to prevent the development of an acute hypertensive emergency. It may also reverse chronic changes from excessive catecholamine stimulation. Pilocarpine is a direct cholinergic agonist. It causes contraction of the smooth muscle of the iris (miosis) and ciliary muscle (accommodation). This causes the iris to retract from the angle of the anterior chamber, followed by opening of the trabecular meshwork at the base of the ciliary muscle. Outflow of aqueous humor occurs into the canal of Schlemm. Acute angle-closure glaucoma eventually requires surgical intervention, but initial therapy could involve a combination of a direct muscarinic agonist (pilocarpine) and a cholinesterase inhibitor (physostigmine)

333–335. The answers are 333-c, 334-a, 335-d. *(Katzung, pp 77–80. Hardman, pp 116, 132, 147–148.)* Acetylcholine is synthesized from acetyl-CoA and choline. Choline is taken up into the neurons by an active transport system. Hemicholinium blocks this uptake, depleting cellular choline, so that synthesis of ACh no longer occurs.

Botulinus toxin comes from *Clostridium botulinum,* an organism that causes food poisoning. Botulinus toxin prevents the release of ACh from nerve endings by mechanisms that are not clear. Death occurs from respiratory failure caused by the inability of diaphragm muscles to contract.

Muscarine, an alkaloid from certain species of mushrooms, is a muscarinic receptor agonist. The compound has toxicologic importance: muscarine poisoning will produce all of the effects that are associated with an overdose of ACh (e.g., bronchoconstriction, bradycardia, hypotension, excessive salivary and respiratory secretion, and sweating). Poisoning by muscarine is treated with atropine.

Local Control Substances

✓Histamine-receptor Antagonists
✓Serotonin agonists
✓Serotonin antagonists
  Ergot alkaloids

✓Prostaglandins and related
  eicosanoids
✓Inhibitors of eicosanoid biosynthesis (NSAIDs)

Questions

DIRECTIONS: Each item below contains a question or incomplete statement followed by suggested responses. Select the **one best** response to each question.

336. Sumatriptan succinate is effective for the treatment of acute migraine headaches by acting as

a. An antagonist at β_1- and β_2-adrenergic receptors
b. A selective antagonist at histamine (H_1) receptors
c. An inhibitor of prostacyclin synthase
d. An agonist at nicotinic receptors
e. A selective agonist at 5-hydroxytryptamine 1D ($5\text{-}HT_{1D}$) receptors

337. Currently, three subtypes of histamine receptors are proposed: H_1 and H_2 receptors are found in peripheral tissues and the central nervous system (CNS), and H_3 receptors are found in the CNS. The second messenger pathway that mediates H_1-receptor stimulation is

a. Increased formation of inositol trisphosphate
b. Elevation of intracellular adenosine $3',5'$-cyclic monophosphate [cyclic AMP (cAMP)]
c. Activation of tyrosine kinases
d. Inhibition of adenylate cyclase activity
e. Activation of sodium (Na^+) ion flow into the cell

338. The pharmacologic effects of acetylsalicylic acid include

- a. Reduction in elevated body temperature
- b. Promotion of platelet aggregation
- c. Alleviation of pain by stimulation of prostaglandin synthesis
- d. Efficacy equal to that of acetaminophen as an anti-inflammatory agent
- e. Less gastric irritation than other salicylates

339. Which of the following is an H_2-receptor antagonist?

- a. Sumatriptan
- b. Cyproheptadine
- c. Ondansetron
- d. Cimetidine
- e. Fluoxetine

340. A 27-year-old male has sprained his ankle, which is swollen and painful, while skiing. X-ray examination is negative except for the appearance of swelling. A nonsteroidal anti-inflammatory drug (NSAID) is administered. Which of the following would be decreased?

- a. Histamine
- b. Cortisol
- c. Bradykinin
- d. Prostacyclin
- e. Uric acid

341. A 74-year-old female has had several episodes of transient ischemic attacks (TIAs). She cannot tolerate aspirin. Which of the following should be considered as an alternative therapy?

- a. Streptokinase
- b. Dipyridamole
- c. Acetaminophen
- d. Ticlopidine
- e. Aminocaproic acid

342. A 16-year-old female is brought to the emergency department (ED) because of increasing drowsiness and inattentiveness. Her family tells you that she takes medication for epilepsy and may have taken an extra dose that day. On examination, she has an ataxic gait, nystagmus, and gingival hypertrophy. What medication does she take?

   a. Phenytoin
   b. Carbamazepine
   c. Ethosuximide
   d. Valproic acid
   e. Trimethadione

343. What is the "on-off phenomenon" that is associated with levodopa (L-dopa) therapy?

   a. Fluctuation in clinical response independent of drug levels
   b. Improvement of clinical response after a drug holiday
   c. Shortened duration of clinical response per dose

344. A 29-year-old female has a 10-year history of migraine headaches. She can usually sense onset. Which of the following agents is the drug of choice for countering acute onset of her headaches?

   a. Ergotamine
   b. Propranolol
   c. Methysergide
   d. Pseudoephedrine
   e. Aspirin

345. Which of the following is a highly selective inhibitor of cyclooxygenase II?

   a. Aspirin
   b. Acetaminophen
   c. Ibuprofen
   d. Celecoxib
   e. Piroxicam

346. A 65-year-old female has swelling and pain in several of the inter-phalangeal (IP) joints of her hand. X-ray examination reveals arthritic changes. Which agent should *not* be prescribed?

   a. Indomethacin
   b. Acetaminophen
   c. Tolmetin
   d. Naproxen
   e. Piroxicam

347. A patient with ulcerative colitis is best treated with

   a. Celecoxib
   b. Naproxen
   c. Sulfasalazine
   d. Infliximab
   e. Penicillamine

348. Which adverse effect of L-dopa therapy is not improved by adding carbidopa?

   a. Mydriasis
   b. Cardiac arrhythmia
   c. Nausea
   d. Depression

349. A 40-year-old male with a diagnosis of moderate to severe asthma is placed on zileuton. What is the mechanism of action of zileuton?

   a. Inhibition of cytokine production
   b. Inhibition of leukotriene production
   c. Inhibition of mediator release
   d. Inhibition of muscarinic receptor action
   e. Inhibition of calcium (Ca^{2+}) channel activity

350. A newborn infant is being prepared for surgical repair of a patent ductus arteriosus. Which of the following agents may be administered pre-operatively?

   a. Zafirleukast
   b. Misoprostol
   c. Timolol
   d. Methysergide
   e. Alprostadil [prostaglandin E_1 (PGE_1)]

Local Control Substances

Answers

336. The answer is e. (*Katzung, pp 280–281.*) Sumatriptan is closely related to serotonin (5-HT) in structure, and it is believed that the drug is effective in the treatment of acute migraine headaches by virtue of its selective agonistic activity at 5-HT$_{1D}$ receptors. These receptors, present on cerebral and meningeal arteries, mediate vasoconstriction induced by 5-HT. In addition, 5-HT$_{1D}$ receptors are found on presynaptic nerve terminals and function to inhibit the release of neuropeptides and other neurotransmitters. It has been suggested that the pain of migraine headaches is caused by vasodilation of intracranial blood vessels and stimulation of trigeminovascular axons, which cause pain and release vasoactive neuropeptides to produce neurogenic inflammation and edema. Sumatriptan acts to reduce vasodilation and the release of neurotransmitters and, therefore, reduces the pain that is associated with migraine headaches. Other antimigraine drugs (e.g., ergotamine and dihydroergotamine) also exhibit high affinities for the 5-HT$_{1D}$-receptor site.

337. The answer is a. (*Katzung, p 267.*) H$_1$ receptors appear to be linked to phospholipase C; activation of these receptors results in an increase in the intracellular formation of inositol-1,4,5-trisphosphate (IP$_3$) and 1,2-diacylglycerol. IP$_3$ binds to a receptor that is located on the endoplasmic reticulum, initiating the release of Ca into the cytosol, where it activates Ca-dependent protein kinases. Diacylglycerol activates protein kinase C. Additionally, stimulation of H$_1$ receptors may activate phospholipase A$_2$ and trigger the arachidonic acid cascade, leading to prostaglandin production.

H$_2$ receptors are associated with adenylate cyclase, and stimulation of these receptors increases the cytosolic concentration of cAMP and activation of cAMP-dependent protein kinase. Although inhibition of adenylate cyclase has been suggested as the intracellular signaling mechanism associated with H$_3$ receptors, this has not been completely substantiated.

338. The answer is a. (*Katzung, pp 599–603.*) Aspirin (acetylsalicylic acid) is the most extensively used analgesic, antipyretic, and anti-inflammatory agent of the group of compounds known as NSAIDs, or nonopioid analgesics. Most of its therapeutic and adverse effects appear to be related to the inhibition of prostaglandin synthesis. Nonsteroidal antiinflammatory drugs inhibit the activity of the enzyme cyclooxygenase, which mediates the conversion of arachidonic acid to prostaglandins that are involved in pain, fever, and inflammation. Aspirin may produce irritation and ulceration of the gastrointestinal (GI) tract, an adverse effect that is about equal to other salicylates. It also inhibits platelet aggregation. Acetaminophen, like aspirin, has analgesic and antipyretic properties, but it does not have clinically significant anti-inflammatory activity and is not irritating to the GI tract.

339. The answer is d. *(Katzung, p 275.)* Cimetidine is an H_2 antagonist that decreases gastric acid secretion. Sumatriptan is a 5-HT$_{1D}$ serotonin agonist. Cyproheptadine acts as a histamine and serotonin antagonist. Ondansetron is a serotonin antagonist. Fluoxetine is an antidepressant agent that selectively inhibits serotonin reuptake.

340. The answer is d. *(Hardman, p 617. Katzung, p 318.)* Most NSAIDs inhibit both cyclooxygenase I and II, resulting in decreased synthesis of prostaglandins, prostacyclins, and thromboxanes.

341. The answer is d. *(Hardman, p 1354. Katzung, pp 574–575.)* Ticlopidine decreases platelet aggregation by inhibiting the uptake of adenosine 5′-diphosphate (ADP) release during degranulation by circulating platelets. Ticlopidine has no effect on prostaglandin synthesis.

342. The answer is a. *(Hardman, pp 469–470.)* Phenytoin has a narrow toxic-therapeutic range. Early signs of phenytoin toxicity are diplopia, nystagmus, and ataxia; sedation occurs at higher drug levels. Gingival hypertrophy, hirsutism, peripheral neuropathy, and folate-deficiency anemia can occur with long-term use. Phenytoin toxicity can be induced by drugs that displace it from plasma proteins.

343. The answer is a. *(Hardman, p 510. Katzung, p 467.)* Fluctuations in clinical response to l-dopa may or may not be related to drug levels (time of last dose). The likelihood of both kinds of fluctuation increases with longer duration of treatment. When these fluctuations are unrelated to drug levels, they are termed the *on-off phenomenon;* the mechanism is unclear.

344. The answer is a. *(Hardman, p 495.)* Ergotamine has several pharmacologic properties, including the blockade of α-adrenergic receptors; however, its mechanism of action in treating migraine headaches is primarily related to its agonistic interaction with serotonin receptors (5-HT_{1D}), resulting in vasoconstriction. Although chronic treatment with this nonsedative, nonanalgesic drug does not decrease the frequency of or prevent migraine attacks, an oral dose of ergotamine is the drug of choice for combating an incipient attack of migraine headache, especially during the prodromal stage.

345. The answer is d. *(Katzung, p 603.)* Celocoxib is a cyclooxygenase-II inhibitor. Aspirin, ibuprofen, and piroxicam are relatively nonselective inhibitors of cyclooxygenases. Acetaminophen has no effect on cyclooxygenases.

346. The answer is b. *(Hardman, pp 631–633.)* All of the drugs listed, except acetaminophen, are usually considered NSAIDs, a large group of structurally dissimilar compounds. These drugs share the pharmacologic properties of the prototype compound, aspirin, in that all have analgesic, antipyretic, and anti-inflammatory effects. The mechanism of action that is responsible for the effect of NSAIDs is reduction in the formation of eicosanoids (e.g., prostaglandins, thromboxanes) by inhibiting the enzyme cyclooxygenase. Acetaminophen differs from the other drugs in that it is a very weak anti-inflammatory agent; however, it is an effective analgesic and antipyretic.

347. The answer is c. *(Katzung, pp 612, 1073.)* Sulfasalazine is a derivative of sulfapyridine and 5-aminosalicylic acid. It is not significantly absorbed following oral administration. The 5-aminosalicyclic acid moiety is released by intestinal bacterial action. Sulfasalazine is more effective in maintaining than causing remission in ulcerative colitis. Celocoxib (a selective cyclooxygenase inhibitor), infliximab (a chimeric monoclonal antibody), and penicillamine (an analogue of cysteine) have a role in the treatment of rheumatoid arthritis. Naproxen, a nonselective cyclooxygenase inhibitor, is indicated for usual rheumatological indications.

348. The answer is d. (*Katzung, pp 464–467.*) Adding carbidopa decreases the amount of dopamine that is formed peripherally from dopa by dopa decarboxylase. Depression, psychosis, and other psychiatric adverse effects of L-dopa are mediated by CNS dopamine, so adding carbidopa does not make them less likely. The combination of L-dopa and carbidopa reduces the extracerebral metabolism of L-dopa, resulting in decreased peripheral adverse effects.

349. The answer is b. (*Katzung, p 344.*) Zileuton is a 5-lipoxygenase inhibitor. Although it is not clear that leukotrienes are partly responsible for the symptoms of asthma, zileuton has a bronchodilator effect that is therapeutically efficacious. The 5-lipoxygenase inhibitors may be less effective than inhaled steroids, but they have the advantage that they are orally administered. This may be an advantage for those individuals who either reject steroid therapy or have difficulty using an inhaler.

350. The answer is e. (*Hardman, p 611.*) Alprostadil [prostaglandin E_1 (PGE_1)] is used therapeutically in preterm infants to temporarily maintain the patency of the ductus arteriosus until corrective surgery can be performed. The drug is administered by continuous intravenous infusion or by catheter through the umbilical artery and should only be used in pediatric intensive care facilities. Misoprostol is a synthetic analogue of PGE_1 (15-deoxy-16-hydroxy-16-methyl-PGE_1 methyl ester). It is indicated for the prevention of gastric ulcers in patients taking NSAIDs (e.g., aspirin, indomethacin) and is administered orally. Zafirleukast is a leukotriene receptor inhibitor, which can be used in asthma. Methysergide is an ergot alkaloid and is used for prophylaxis in patients with migraine headaches. Timolol is a β-adrenergic antagonist that is useful in the treatment of glaucoma.

Renal System

Carbonic anhydrase inhibitors
Loop diuretics
Osmotic diuretics
Potassium (K^+)-sparing diuretics

Thiazides (benzodiathiazide)
    diuretics
Antidiuretic hormone

Questions

DIRECTIONS: Each item below contains a question or incomplete statement followed by suggested responses. Select the **one best** response to each question.

351. Of the following agents, which is best avoided in a patient with a history of chronic congestive heart failure (CHF)?

a. Hydrochlorothiazide
b. Amiloride
c. Mannitol
d. Ethacrynic acid
e. Spironolactone

352. Furosemide inhibits the sodium-potassium-dichloride (Na^+, K^+, $2Cl_2^-$) co-transporters that are located in the

a. Collecting duct
b. Ascending limb of the loop of Henle
c. Descending limb of the loop of Henle
d. Proximal tubule
e. Distal convoluted tubule

353. Of the following agents, which is best avoided when a patient is being treated with an aminoglycoside?

a. Metolazone
b. Triamterene
c. Furosemide
d. Spironolactone
e. Acetazolamide

354. Hyperkalemia is a contraindication to the use of which of the following drugs?

a. Acetazolamide
b. Chlorothiazide
c. Ethacrynic acid
d. Chlorthalidone
e. Spironolactone

355. A reduction in insulin release from the pancreas may be caused by which of the following diuretics?

a. Triamterene
b. Chlorothiazide
c. Spironolactone
d. Acetazolamide
e. Amiloride

356. Acute uric acid nephropathy, which is characterized by the acute overproduction of uric acid and by extreme hyperuricemia, can best be prevented with which of the following?

a. Antidiuretic hormone (ADH) [vasopressin (VP)]
b. Cyclophosphamide
c. Allopurinol
d. Amiloride
e. Sodium chloride (NaCl)

357. The release of ADH is suppressed by which of the following drugs to promote a diuresis?

a. Guanethidine
b. Acetazolamide
c. Chlorothiazide
d. Ethanol
e. Indomethacin

358. Conservation of K ions in the body occurs with which of the following diuretics?

a. Furosemide
b. Hydrochlorothiazide
c. Triamterene
d. Metolazone
e. Bumetanide

359. Spironolactone can be characterized by which one of the following statements?

a. It is biotransformed to an inactive product
b. It binds to a cytoplasmic receptor
c. It is a more potent diuretic than is hydrochlorothiazide
d. It interferes with aldosterone synthesis
e. It inhibits Na reabsorption in the proximal renal tubule of the nephron

360. Which of the following diuretics could be added to the therapeutic regimen of a patient who is receiving a direct vasodilator for the treatment of hypertension?

a. Acetazolamide
b. Triamterene
c. Spironolactone
d. Mannitol
e. Hydrochlorothiazide

361. A patient develops acute gout following treatment with which of the following?

a. Acetazolamide
b. Allopurinol
c. Triamterene
d. Spironolactone
e. Furosemide

362. A patient with nephrogenic diabetes insipidus is best treated with which of the following?

a. Hydrochlorothiazide
b. Triamterene
c. Furosemide
d. Spironolactone
e. Acetazolamide

363. Which of the following is unlikely to cause a drug-drug interaction with the thiazides?

a. Adrenal corticosteroids
b. Anticoagulants (oral)
c. Aminoglycosides
d. Uricosuric agents
e. Insulin

364. Of the following diuretic agents, which would be least likely to indirectly cause an increased binding of digoxin to cardiac tissue sodium–potassium–adenosine triphosphatase ($Na^+, K^+, ATPase$)?

a. Hydrochlorothiazide
b. Furosemide
c. Amiloride
d. Acetazolamide
e. Metolazone

365. A patient with compromised renal hemodynamics is given a trial of mannitol. Of the following, which is the least likely to be associated with the effect of mannitol?

a. Retention of water in the tubular fluid
b. Ability to be metabolically altered to an active form
c. Capacity to be freely filtered
d. Effectiveness as nonelectrolytic, osmotically active particles
e. Ability to resist complete reabsorption by the renal tubule

366. A patient develops hyperglycemia, hyperuricemia, and hypomagnesemia on which of the following diuretic agents?

a. Hydrochlorothiazide
b. Triamterene
c. Spironolactone
d. Acetazolamide
e. Amiloride

367. Of the following, which adverse reaction is not associated with furosemide?

a. Hyperglycemia
b. Tinnitus
c. Fluid and electrolyte imbalance
d. Hypotension
e. Metabolic acidosis

368. A 35-year-old male has renal stones and increased calcium (Ca) in the urine that is associated with normal serum Ca and parathyroid hormone levels. Which of the following agents could be used to treat this patient?

a. Furosemide
b. Acetazolamide
c. Triamterene
d. Hydrochlorothiazide
e. Vasopressin

369. In which of the following are thiazide diuretics ineffective?

a. Edema caused by CHF
b. Edema induced by glucocorticoids
c. Hypertension with or without edema
d. Ascites
e. Glaucoma

Questions 370–372

The figure below shows proposed sites of action of drugs. For each of the diuretic agents below, choose the anatomic site in the schematic diagram of the renal nephron where the principal action of the agent occurs.

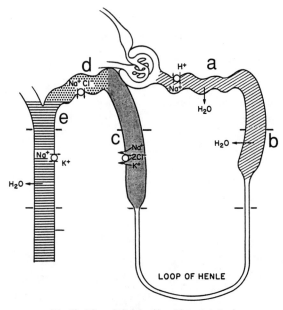

(Modified from DiPalma, 4/e, with permission.)

370. Ethacrynic acid

371. Hydrochlorothiazide

372. Triamterene

Questions 373–375

The table below shows the urinary excretion patterns of electrolytes of diuretic drugs. For each of the diuretic agents listed below, choose the urinary excretion pattern that the drug would produce.

Drug	Na$^+$	Cl$^-$	K$^+$	Ca^{2+}	HCO$_3^-$	Mg^{2+}
a.	+	+	+	−	±	+
b.	+	+	+	−	0	+
c.	+	+	+	+	0	+
d.	+	+	−	0	+	0
e.	+	−	+	0	+	0

+, increase; −, decrease; 0, no change; ±, increase dependent on dose.

373. Triamterene

374. Furosemide

375. Hydrochlorothiazide

376. Which of the following decreases the urinary excretion of Cl ions?

a. Chlorthalidone
b. Triamterene
c. Acetazolamide
d. Furosemide
e. Mannitol

377. A 50-year-male with pitting edema of the ankles develops gynecomastia and erectile dysfunction while being treated with which of the following agents?

a. Hydrochlorothiazide
b. Metolazone
c. Spironolactone
d. Triamterene
e. Amiloride

378. A 55-year-old female with a blood pressure of 170/105 mmHg has pitting edema of the lower extremities and an elevated serum creatinine associated with a normal serum potassium. Which of the following agents is contraindicated in this patient?

a. Triamterene
b. Hydrochlorothiazide
c. Metolazone
d. Ethacrynic acid
e. Acetazolamide

379. A 60-year-old male with an uncontrolled blood pressure of 170/105 mmHg is treated with enalapril. What is the mechanism of action of enalapril?

a. α-adrenergic receptor agonist
b. α-adrenergic receptor antagonist
c. β-adrenergic receptor agonist
d. β-adrenergic receptor antagonist
e. Ganglionic blocking agent
f. Depletion of nerve terminal storage of norepinephrine (NE)
g. Direct smooth-muscle vasodilator
h. Angiotensin converting enzyme (ACE) antagonist
i. Angiotensin receptor antagonist

380. A 75-year-old female with a blood pressure of 180/95 mmHg is treated with terazosin. What is the mechanism of action of terazosin?

a. α-adrenergic receptor agonist
b. α-adrenergic receptor antagonist
c. β-adrenergic receptor agonist
d. β-adrenergic receptor antagonist
e. Ganglionic blocking agent
f. Depletion of nerve terminal storage of NE
g. Direct smooth-muscle vasodilator
h. ACE antagonist
i. Angiotensin receptor antagonist

381. A 50-year-old male is seen in the emergency department (ED) with a blood pressure of 260/160 mmHg. Blurring optic discs with indistinct margins are seen on ophthalmologic examination. An intravenous drip of sodium nitroprusside is administered. What is the mechanism of action of sodium nitroprusside?

a. α-adrenergic receptor agonist
b. α-adrenergic receptor antagonist
c. β-adrenergic receptor agonist
d. β-adrenergic receptor antagonist
e. Ganglionic blocking agent
f. Depletion of nerve terminal storage of NE
g. Direct smooth-muscle vasodilator
h. ACE antagonist
i. Angiotensin receptor antagonist

Renal System

Answers

351. The answer is c. *(Hardman, pp 695–697.)* Mannitol increases serum osmolarity and therefore pulls water out of cells, cerebrospinal fluid (CSF), and aqueous humor. This effect can be useful in the treatment of elevated intraocular or intracranial pressure. However, by expanding the intravascular volume, mannitol can exacerbate CHF.

352. The answer is b. *(Katzung, pp 252–254.)* Furosemide is a loop diuretic that promotes the urinary excretion of Na and Cl. This diuretic agent blocks the reabsorption of Na and Cl by inhibiting the Na^+, K^+, $2Cl^-$ co-transporters in the ascending limb of the loop of Henle. Although this co-transport mechanism requires energy from converting adenosine triphosphate (ATP) to adenosine 5′-diphosphate (ADP) by Na^+,K^+,ATPase, furosemide does not directly inhibit the enzyme Na^+,K^+,ATPase. Along with the net loss of Na and Cl^-, loop diuretics produce an increase in the urinary excretion of Ca and Mg by interfering with the reabsorption of these ions in the ascending limb of the loop of Henle. In addition, furosemide, like the other loop diuretic agents, can cause hypokalemia. The secretion of the K occurs as a consequence of the reabsorption of Na in the late distal convoluted tubule and the collecting duct.

353. The answer is c. *(Hardman, p 700. Katzung, pp 785–786.)* The loop diuretic furosemide is an example of a drug that can cause several drug-drug interactions. Because the loop diuretic can cause hearing impairment, it can augment the ototoxicity that can occur with other drugs, such as aminoglycoside antibiotics (e.g., gentamicin, streptomycin, tobramycin). Furosemide undergoes proximal tubule secretion. This renal secretory mechanism, which is associated with renal excretion, is also available to a number of organic acids, such as the salicylates. When salicylates are present in the body, furosemide is a competitive inhibitor of their excretion by this particular mechanism in the proximal tubule; therefore, the plasma levels of salicylates are increased with the potential for adverse reactions in the patient. Furosemide can enhance the toxicity of lithium by reducing its renal excretion.

354. The answer is e. (*Hardman, p 708.*) Spironolactone is a competitive antagonist of aldosterone that blocks the reabsorption of Na and water from the collecting duct in exchange for K and hydrogen ion retention. Therefore, in the presence of hyperkalemia, spironolactone is contraindicated. The administration of each of the other diuretic agents listed results in increased excretion of K.

355. The answer is b. (*Hardman, pp 702–704.*) An adverse reaction that is reported to occur occasionally with the thiazides, such as chlorothiazide, is hyperglycemia. In addition, hyperglycemia may occur with thiazide-related compounds (chlorthalidone and metolazone) and the high-ceiling diuretics (ethacrynic acid, furosemide, and bumetanide). The proposed mechanism for the elevation in blood glucose appears to be related to a decrease in insulin release from the pancreas. In addition, increased glycogenolysis, decreased glycogenesis, and a reduction in the conversion of proinsulin to insulin may also be involved in the hyperglycemic response. Diazoxide, a nondiuretic thiazide, is given to treat hypoglycemia in certain conditions. However, diazoxide is used more often to control hypertensive emergencies.

356. The answer is c. (*Hardman, pp 649–650.*) Acute hyperuricemia, which often occurs in patients who are treated with cytotoxic drugs for neoplasic disorders, can lead to the deposition of urate crystals in the kidneys and their collecting ducts. This can produce partial or complete obstruction of the collecting ducts, renal pelvis, or ureter. Allopurinol and its primary metabolite, alloxanthine, are inhibitors of xanthine oxidase, an enzyme that catalyzes the oxidation of hypoxanthine and xanthine to uric acid. The use of allopurinol in patients at risk can markedly reduce the likelihood that they will develop acute uric acid nephropathy.

357. The answer is d. (*Hardman, p 721.*) Ethanol produces a diuretic response by inhibiting the release of ADH from the posterior pituitary gland. Less ADH acts on the collecting duct of the nephron and, therefore, the amount of water reabsorbed by the collecting duct is reduced. Indomethacin enhances the release of ADH, which increases the permeability of the collecting duct to water. Acetazolamide and chlorothiazide promote a diuresis by acting on a site directly in the nephron unit to reduce the reabsorption of NaCl and water. Guanethidine, an antihypertensive agent, does not appear to alter the release of ADH.

358. The answer is c. (Hardman, pp 704–706.) Triamterene produces retention of the K ion by inhibiting in the collecting duct the reabsorption of Na, which is accompanied by the excretion of K ions. The loop diuretics furosemide and bumetanide cause as a possible adverse action the development of hypokalemia. In addition, thiazides (e.g., hydrochlorothiazide) and the thiazide-related agents (e.g., metolazone) can cause the loss of K ions with the consequences of hypokalemia. Triamterene can be given with a loop diuretic or thiazide to prevent or correct the condition of hypokalemia.

359. The answer is b. (Hardman, pp 706–709.) Spironolactone is a K-sparing diuretic. The drug is well absorbed from the gastrointestinal tract and is biotransformed in the liver to an active metabolite, canrenone. Spironolactone is contraindicated in the presence of hyperkalemia, because this aldosterone antagonist may cause further elevation of plasma K concentrations. It does not appear to depress adrenal or pituitary function. Central nervous system (CNS) side effects of the drug can include lethargy, headache, drowsiness, and mental confusion. Spironolactone displaces aldosterone from receptor sites that are responsible for Na resorption in the collecting duct of the nephron; it does not interfere with the synthesis of aldosterone.

360. The answer is e. (Hardman, pp 701, 704, 706, 708, 783, 795. Katzung, p 169.) Patients treated with direct vasodilators develop significant volume retention. In decreasing arterial pressure, direct vasodilators decrease renal sodium excretion and increase aldosterone secretion. These effects are blocked by thiazide diuretics. In addition, in the treatment of essential hypertension, even without obvious edema, thiazides exert a hypotensive action that has proven beneficial. Furosemide usually is administered with minoxidil because of its association with salt and water retention, compared with hydralazine. The carbonic anhydrase inhibitor acetazolamide, by inhibiting the secretion of aqueous humor, has the property of decreasing intraocular pressure—an effect of value for patients who have glaucoma. Triamterene and spironolactone may have beneficial effects in the treatment of chronic CHF but are generally used in combination with the thiazides, particularly with the objective of minimally disturbing K homeostasis.

361. The answer is e. (Katzung, p 254.) Furosemide affects the reabsorption of uric acid in the proximal tubule. It increases uric acid reabsorption because of its capacity to produce significant hypovolemia. The ensuing hyperuricemia can lead to acute attacks of gout.

362. The answer is a. *(Katzung, pp 255–256.)* Thiazide diuretics can be used in the treatment of nephrogenic diabetes insipidus. Its other uses include the treatment of hypertension, CHF, and nephrolithiasis due to idiopathic hypercalcuria.

363. The answer is c. *(Hardman, 650, 702–703.)* Drug interactions are reported for various drugs and the thiazide diuretics. Thiazides can indirectly promote the loss of K from the collecting duct of the nephron, and adrenal corticosteroids can enhance the hypokalemic effect. A lethal drug interaction of the thiazides with quinidine leading to polymorphic tachycardia may result from thiazide-induced hypokalemia. The therapeutic effect of oral anticoagulants may be reduced by thiazides because these diuretics can concentrate clotting factors in the blood. Thiazides elevate plasma urate levels, perhaps counteracting the effects of uricosuric agents. The combination of allopurinol and thiazides in patients with compromised renal function has resulted in hypersensitivity reactions. In addition, the neuromuscular blocking action of tubocurarine is enhanced by thiazide diuretics. Aminoglycosides, which can cause eighth-nerve damage, can increase the ototoxicity that is associated with the use of the loop diuretics. Tinnitus and ototoxicity have not been reported as adverse reactions for the thiazide diuretics.

364. The answer is c. *(Katzung, pp 249–258.)* Diuretic therapy can lead to the development of hypokalemia. The thiazides (hydrochlorothiazide), thiazide-related compounds (metolazone), the proximal tubule diuretics (acetazolamide), and loop diuretics (furosemide) can produce the loss of K from the blood through the late distal tubule and collecting duct into the renal tubular fluid. When any of these drugs are administered in the presence of digitalis glycoside (digoxin), there is the potential for digitalis toxicities to occur. The development of these toxicities is related to the fact that in the presence of hypokalemia there is greater affinity of digitalis glycosides to cardiac tissue $Na^+,K^+,ATPase$. However, when the hypokalemia is corrected and the plasma levels of K are returned toward normal, digitalis toxicities are usually eliminated. Triamterene, which is a K-sparing diuretic, does not cause hypokalemia and, therefore, would not enhance the binding of digoxin to

Na^+,K^+,ATPase. It also promotes the conservation of K and can cause the adverse reaction of hyperkalemia.

365. The answer is b. *(Hardman, pp 695–697.)* A significant increase in the amount of any osmotically active solute in voided urine is usually accompanied by an increase in urine volume. Osmotic diuretics affect diuresis through this principle. The osmotic diuretics (such as mannitol) are nonelectrolytes that are freely filtered at the glomerulus, undergo limited reabsorption by the renal tubules, retain water in the renal tubule, and promote an osmotic diuresis, generally without significant Na excretion. In addition, these diuretics resist alteration by metabolic processes.

366. The answer is a. *(Hardman, pp 700–702. Katzung, pp 252–256.)* The thiazide diuretics and the loop diuretics have a number of adverse reactions in common. Hydrochlorothiazide and the loop diuretics cause hyperglycemia by possibly reducing the secretion of insulin from the pancreas. Because these drugs can elevate blood levels of glucose, they should be used with caution when administered to patients with diabetes mellitus. The development of hyperuricemia as a consequence of the use of hydrochlorothiazide or loop diuretics is related to the fact that these drugs interfere with the proximal tubule secretion of uric acid because of volume depletion. The alteration in serum Mg (hypomagnesemia) is caused by both hydrochlorothiazide and the loop diuretics, by blocking the reabsorption of Mg.

367. The answer is e. *(Hardman, pp 697–701.)* The loop, or high-ceiling, diuretics furosemide and ethacrynic acid are cleared by the kidney with such celerity that even high doses repeatedly administered do not result in significant accumulation. Chronic administration of these agents, however, may lead to alkalosis with hyponatremia in association with rapid removal of edema fluid. Other toxic manifestations of loop diuretics include fluid and electrolyte imbalance, gastrointestinal symptoms, interstitial nephritis, hyperglycemia, tinnitus, and infrequent, but serious, ototoxicity. Besides being used as a diuretic agent, furosemide is used in the treatment of hypertension.

368. The answer is d. *(Hardman, pp 701–702, 704. Katzung, p 741.)* Hydrochlorothiazide is recommended in the treatment of idiopathic hypercalciuria because of its ability to decrease the excretion of Ca. The loop diuretics are contraindicated because they increase urinary Ca excretion. The mechanism for decreased Ca excretion by the thiazides is not known, but it is thought that inhibition of NaCl co-transport in the distal tubules by thiazides causes membrane depolarization. This results in the opening of the Ca channels followed by the reabsorption of Ca.

369. The answer is e. *(Katzung, pp 255–256.)* Thiazides are most useful as diuretic agents in the management of edema caused by chronic cardiac decompensation. In the treatment of hypertensive disease, even without obvious edema, thiazides exert a hypotensive action that has proved beneficial. Less common uses of thiazide diuretics include the treatment of edema from glucocorticoids, diabetes insipidus, and hypercalciuria. The carbonic anhydrase inhibitor acetazolamide, by inhibiting the secretion of aqueous humor, has the property of decreasing intraocular pressure—a valuable effect for patients who have glaucoma.

370–372. The answers are 370-c, 371-d, 372-e. *(Hardman, pp 697, 701, 705.)* The loop diuretic ethacrynic acid has its site of action in the ascending limb of the loop of Henle. This drug inhibits the reabsorption of Na and Cl^- by interfering with the Na^+, K^+, $2Cl^-$ co-transport system. In addition, loop diuretics block the reabsorption of Mg and Ca from the renal tubular fluid into the blood in this segment of the nephron unit.

Hydrochlorothiazide has its proposed site of action at the distal convoluted tubule or, more specifically, at the early portion of the distal tubule. Hydrochlorothiazide inhibits the reabsorption of Na and Cl. It also promotes the reabsorption of Ca back into the blood, but inhibits the reabsorption of Mg from the renal tubular fluid. The K-sparing diuretic agents (spironolactone, triamterene, and amiloride) have their site of action in the nephron at the late distal tubule and the collecting duct. These diuretic agents only cause a mild natriuretic effect.

373–375. The answers are 373-d, 374-c, 375-a. *(Katzung, pp 253–254, 256–257.)* The urinary excretion pattern of electrolytes for the thiazide diuretic agents (e.g., hydrochlorothiazide) shown in the table that accompanies the question is represented by choice a. These drugs block the reabsorption of Na and Cl at the early distal convoluted tubule of the nephron. In addition, they promote the excretion of K and Mg. At high doses, the thiazide diuretics (especially hydrochlorothiazide) may cause a slight increase in bicarbonate excretion. As for the Ca ion, the thiazide diuretic agents enhance the distal tubular reabsorption of Ca, and, therefore, Ca urinary excretion may decrease. The loop diuretics (bumetanide, furosemide, ethacrynic acid) are the most potent group of diuretics. These drugs act at the ascending limb of the loop of Henle and interfere with the co-transport of Na and Cl. In addition, they cause the excretion of K, Mg, and Ca into the urine.

The K-sparing group of diuretics produce their diuretic response by reduction of the reabsorption of Na in the later distal convoluted tubule and the collecting duct. They cause an increase in the urinary excretion of NaCl and possibly bicarbonate, while they reduce the excretion of K. The K-sparing diuretic agents do not appear to have any significant effect on the excretion of Mg and Ca ions.

376. The answer is c. (*Hardman, pp 691, 693.*) Acetazolamide is a carbonic anhydrase inhibitor with its primary site of action at the proximal tubule of the nephron. Acetazolamide promotes a urinary excretion of Na, K, and bicarbonate. There is a decrease in loss of Cl⁻ ions. The increased excretion of bicarbonate makes the urine alkaline and may produce metabolic acidosis as a consequence of the loss of bicarbonate from the blood. None of the other diuretic drugs promote a reduction in the excretion of the Cl⁻ ion.

377. The answer is c. (*Hardman, pp 706–708.*) Spironolactone is an aldosterone antagonist that acts on the mineralocorticoid receptor. It is a K-sparing diuretic. It can also function as an androgen antagonist, which could explain the gynecomastia and erectile dysfunction. Women with hirsutism are sometimes treated with spironolactone.

378. The answer is a. (*Hardman, pp 705–706.*) Patients at increased risk of developing hyperkalemia should not receive K-sparing diuretics. Potassium-sparing diuretics appear to block Na channels in the luminal membrane of the late distal tubules and the collecting duct. A mild excretion of Na occurs because of the relatively low capacity to reabsorb it in this portion of the nephron. Loop diuretics and thiazides typically increase K excretion.

379. The answer is h. (*Katzung, pp 172–174.*) Enalapril is converted to its active form by de-esterification to enalaprilat, which is capable of inhibiting the ACE, peptidyl peptidase. Levels of bradykinin also increase because of inhibition of the enzyme. Bradykinin can stimulate the release of nitric oxide. It is thought that the lowering of blood pressure by enalapril is due to both its inhibitory effect on the renin-angiotensin system and its stimulation of the kallikrein-kinin system.

380. The answer is b. *(Hardman, p 229. Katzung, p 168.)* Terazosin blocks α receptors in arterioles and venules. It is $α_1$-selective. Perhaps this selectivity permits NE to exert unopposed negative feedback on its own release because of little or no effect on presynaptic $α_2$ receptors. Alpha blockers reduce arterial pressure in both resistance and capacitance vessels and, therefore, are quite effective in reducing blood pressure when a patient is in the upright position.

381. The answer is g. *(Katzung, pp 170–171.)* Sodium nitroprusside reduces blood pressure by dilating both arterial and venous vessels. It most likely acts by releasing nitric oxide, which reacts with guanylyl cyclase. This results in an increase in intracellular cyclic guanosine 5′-monophosphate [cyclic GMP (cGMP)], a vascular smooth-muscle relaxant. Another possible explanation for increased intracellular levels of GMP is the direct action of sodium nitroprusside on guanylyl cyclase. Sodium nitroprusside is a useful agent in the treatment of hypertensive emergencies because of its rapid onset and short duration of action.

Gastrointestinal System and Nutrition

Antacids
Histamine-2 (H$_2$)-receptor antagonists
Muscarinic receptor antagonists
Proton-pump inhibitors
Mucosal protective agents
Pancreatic replacement enzymes
Laxatives

Antidiarrheals
Agents for dissolution of gallstones
Agents for inflammatory bowel disease
Agents for portal system encephalopathy
Vitamins

Questions

DIRECTIONS: Each item below contains a question or incomplete statement followed by suggested responses. Select the **one best** response to each question.

382. Cimetidine slows the metabolism of many drugs because it inhibits the activity of

a. Monoamine oxidase (MAO)
b. Cytochrome P450
c. Tyrosine kinase
d. Hydrogen–potassium–adenosine triphosphatase (H$^+$,K$^+$,ATPase)
e. Phase II glucuronidation reactions

383. The absorption of phosphate is reduced when large and prolonged doses of which of the following antacids are given?
a. Na bicarbonate
b. Mg hydroxide
c. Mg trisilicate
d. Ca carbonate
e. Sucralfate

384. Omeprazole, an agent for the promotion of healing of peptic ulcers, has a mechanism of action that is based on

a. Prostaglandins
b. Gastric secretion
c. Pepsin secretion
d. H$^+$,K$^+$,ATPase
e. Anticholinergic action

385. An effective antidiarrheal agent that inhibits peristaltic movement is

a. Clonidine
b. Bismuth subsalicylate
c. Oral electrolyte solution
d. Atropine
e. Diphenoxylate

386. The approved indication for misoprostol

a. Reflux esophagitis
b. Regional ileitis
c. Ulcerative colitis
d. Prevention of gastric ulceration in patients using large doses of aspirin-like drugs
e. Pathologic hypersecretory conditions such as Zollinger-Ellison syndrome

387. Metoclopramide has antiemetic properties because it

a. Accelerates gastric emptying time
b. Lowers esophageal sphincter pressure
c. Is a central nervous system (CNS) dopamine-receptor antagonist
d. Has cholinomimetic properties
e. Has sedative properties

388. The steatorrhea of pancreatic insufficiency can best be treated by

a. Cimetidine
b. Misoprostol
c. Bile salts
d. Pancrelipase
e. Secretin

389. Cholesterol gallstones may be dissolved by oral treatment with

a. Lovastatin
b. Dehydrocholic acid
c. Methyl tertiary butyl ether
d. Chenodeoxycholic acid
e. Monoctanoin

390. A drug of choice in the therapy of inflammatory bowel disease is

a. Sulfadiazine
b. Sulfasalazine
c. Sulfapyridine
d. Sulfamethoxazole
e. Salicylate sodium

391. An important drug in the therapy of portal systemic encephalopathy is

a. Lactulose
b. Lactate
c. Loperamide
d. Lorazepam
e. Loxapine

392. Bismuth salts are thought to be effective in peptic ulcer disease because they have bactericidal properties against

a. *Escherichia coli*
b. *Bacteroides fragilis*
c. *Clostridium difficile*
d. *Helicobacter pylori*
e. *Staphylococcus aureus*

393. Misoprostol has a cytoprotective action on the gastrointestinal (GI) mucosa because it

a. Enhances secretion of mucus and bicarbonate ion
b. Neutralizes acid secretion
c. Antagonizes nonsteroidal anti-inflammatory drugs (NSAIDs)
d. Relieves ulcer symptoms
e. Coats the mucosa

394. For the severe form of nodulocystic acne vulgaris, the first line of therapy is the systemic use of

a. Vitamin A
b. Retinol
c. Tetracycline
d. Isotretinoin (13-*cis*-retinoic acid)
e. Ciprofloxacin

395. The primary pharmacologic action of omeprazole is the reduction of

a. Volume of gastric juice
b. Gastric motility
c. Secretion of pepsin
d. Secretion of gastric acid
e. Secretion of intrinsic factor

396. Which of the following vitamins in large doses is teratogenic?

a. Vitamin A
b. Vitamin B_{12}
c. Vitamin C
d. Vitamin D
e. Vitamin E

397. Fat-soluble vitamins generally have a greater potential toxicity compared with water-soluble vitamins because they are

a. More essential to vital metabolic processes
b. Metabolically faster
c. Avidly stored by the body
d. Administered in larger doses
e. Involved in more essential metabolic pathways

398. In the United States, the recommended daily allowances (RDAs) are periodically developed by the

a. National Research Council (NRC)
b. Food and Drug Administration (FDA)
c. Department of Agriculture
d. Department of Commerce
e. Surgeon General

399. Which vitamin needs to be given in supplemental doses in order to prevent deficiency when a patient is given prolonged administration of isoniazid (INH)?

a. Vitamin A
b. Vitamin K
c. Vitamin C
d. Thiamine
e. Pyridoxine

400. Which of the following is a stool softener that has no effect on absorption of fat-soluble vitamins?

a. Mineral oil
b. Castor oil
c. Docusate sodium
d. Phenolphthalein
e. Cascara sagrada

401. Which of the following is not associated with sucralfate?

a. It contains polyaluminum hydroxide
b. It maintains gellike qualities even at acid pH
c. It binds to ulcer craters more than to normal mucosae
d. It has moderate acid-neutralizing properties
e. It reacts very little with mucin

DIRECTIONS: Each group of questions below consists of lettered options followed by a set of numbered items. For each numbered item, select the **one** lettered option with which it is **most** closely associated. Each lettered option may be used once, more than once, or not at all.

Questions 402–403

Match each vitamin with the appropriate description.

a. Excess amounts should be avoided when the patient is on levodopa (L-dopa)
b. Overdosage may lead to a psychotic state
c. Improvement of vision especially in daylight might be attributable to this vitamin
d. This vitamin is usually not included in the popular one-a-day vitamin preparations
e. Retinoic acid is the natural form
f. Acute intoxication with this vitamin causes hypertension, nausea, and vomiting, and signs of increased cerebrospinal fluid (CSF) pressure
g. This vitamin has hormonal functions
h. This fat-soluble vitamin has mainly antioxidant properties
i. In its water-soluble form, this fat-soluble vitamin is capable of producing kernicterus

402. Calcitriol (vitamin D metabolite—1,25-dihydroxyvitamin D)

403. Pyridoxine

Questions 404–405

For each vitamin, match the appropriate use or deficiency.

a. Large doses are used to treat hyperlipoproteinemia
b. Large doses are used to acidify urine
c. This vitamin is used in the therapy of Wernicke's syndrome
d. Large doses are used to cure psychosis
e. Deficiency can cause angular stomatitis
f. Deficiency can cause the common cold
g. Deficiency can cause convulsions in children

404. Riboflavin

405. Thiamine

Questions 406–407

Match the main therapeutic potential with the correctly listed GI drug.

a. Ranitidine
b. Metronidazole
c. Omeprazole
d. Sucralfate
e. Misoprostol
f. Ca carbonate
g. Loperamide

406. Preferred drug therapy for Zollinger-Ellison syndrome

407. Helpful in selected cases of diarrhea

Questions 408–409

There are different mechanisms by which laxatives achieve their effects. Match the mechanism to the correct drug.

a. Mg sulfate
b. Methylcellulose
c. Phenolphthalein
d. Castor oil
e. Lactulose
f. Mineral oil
g. Docusate Na (dioctyl sodium sulfosuccinate)

408. Has a hyperosmotic mechanism different from that of saline cathartics

409. Increases colonic peristalsis and enhances fluid and electrolyte secretion into the bowel

Questions 410–411

A large number of endogenous and exogenous agents act to alter the rate of acid secretion by the parietal cell. Match the mechanism to the agent.

a. Histamine
b. Gastrin
c. Acetylcholine (ACh)
d. Aspirin
e. Food
f. Al hydroxide
g. Bismuth subsalicylate
h. Omeprazole
i. Misoprostol
j. Sucralfate

410. Lowers gastric secretion and is contraindicated in women of childbearing age

411. Increases gastric acidity by preventing the action of inhibitory guanine nucleotide-binding protein (G protein) on adenylate cyclase

Gastrointestinal System and Nutrition

Answers

382. The answer is b. *(Hardman, p 906.)* Cimetidine reversibly inhibits cytochrome P450. This is important in phase I biotransformation reactions and inhibits the metabolism of such drugs as warfarin, phenytoin, propranolol, metoprolol, quinidine, and theophylline. None of the other enzymes are significantly affected.

383. The answer is d. *(Katzung, pp 1064–1066.)* Although Al hydroxide is generally considered to be the antacid that inhibits phosphate absorption, Ca carbonate is equally capable of this effect. This adverse effect may be hazardous in the presence of renal impairment.

384. The answer is d. *(Hardman, pp 907–909.)* Omeprazole inhibits H^+,K^+,ATPase, which effectively stops the proton pump and thus prevents the formation of gastric acid. It is the most effective agent in severe cases of ulceration and esophageal reflux.

385. The answer is e. *(Hardman, p 926.)* Diphenoxylate is a piperidine opioid that is related to meperidine. It inhibits peristalsis and, hence, increases the passage time of the intestinal bolus. It is combined with atropine to discourage use as a street drug. Atropine has little effect on peristalsis. Clonidine, bismuth subsalicylate, and rehydration therapy are all useful in some types of diarrhea, but none of them inhibit peristalsis.

386. The answer is d. *(Hardman, p 611.)* Misoprostol is a prostaglandin E (PGE) analogue that has antisecretory and mucosal protection properties in the stomach. Experimentally, it protects against mucosal damage from NSAIDs, alcohol, and other toxic agents. It will also tend to heal existing ulcers, but it is inferior to other agents in this regard.

387. The answer is c. *(Hardman, pp 932–933.)* Metoclopramide antagonizes the emetic effect of apomorphine, which is mediated by a dopamine receptor in the CNS. It also raises the lower esophageal sphincter pressure and relaxes the pyloric sphincter, which hastens gastric emptying time. This makes it useful in the therapy of reflux esophagitis.

388. The answer is d. (Hardman, p 935.) Pancrelipase is an alcoholic extract of hog pancreas that contains lipase, trypsin, and amylase. It is effective in reducing the steatorrhea of pancreatic insufficiency. None of the other drugs mentioned have significant action in the digestion of fats.

389. The answer is d. (Hardman, pp 934–935.) Chenodeoxycholic acid (chenodiol) and ursodiol have proved to be effective in some patients with cholesterol gallstones. Lovastatin lowers blood cholesterol levels but has no effect on gallstones. Methyl tertiary butyl ether and a new agent, monoctanoin, are infused directly into the common duct and will dissolve gallstones.

390. The answer is b. (Hardman, p 1061.) Sulfasalazine consists of sulfapyridine with 5-aminosalicylic acid linked by an azo- bond. This bond is broken by bacteria that release the salicylic acid, which is believed to be the active agent. Sulfa drugs or salicylic acid used alone is not as effective. The mechanism of action is unknown, but it is believed to be protective action on the mucosa by inhibition of the synthesis of prostaglandins and leukotrienes.

391. The answer is a. (Hardman, p 922.) Lactulose is a synthetic disaccharide (galactose-fructose) that is not absorbed. In moderate doses, it acts as a laxative. In higher doses, it is capable of binding ammonia and other toxins that form in the intestine in severe liver deficiency and that are believed to cause the encephalopathy. Loperamide is an antidiarrheal opioid; lorazepam is a CNS depressant; loxapine is a heterocyclic antipsychotic.

392. The answer is d. (Hardman, pp 909–910.) It is now recognized that infection with H. pylori is a major etiologic factor in peptic ulcer disease. Bismuth salts are bactericidal for many organisms but especially for spirochetes. Colloidal bismuth salts such as bismuth subsalicylate also have a coating or cytoprotective action. Antimicrobials and GI antisecretory drugs are also used in combination with bismuth compounds.

393. The answer is a. (*Hardman, p 914.*) Misoprostol is a prostaglandin analogue of PGE with an affinity for the gastric mucosa. It stimulates the secretion of mucus and bicarbonate, enhances cell proliferation, preserves the microcirculation, and stabilizes tissue lysosomes. Misoprostol is approved by the FDA for protection against the ulcerogenic action of NSAIDs (not because it antagonizes NSAIDs).

394. The answer is d. (*Hardman, p 1575.*) Isotretinoin is actually a form of high-dose vitamin A therapy. Vitamin A itself or retinol (vitamin A_1) could be used, but they have less advantageous pharmacokinetic properties. Antibiotics such as tetracyclines are used in acne, but they have little effect on the nodulocystic form.

395. The answer is d. (*Hardman, pp 907–909.*) The main action of omeprazole is the inhibition of secretion of gastric acid. Because it is a specific inhibitor of the proton pump ($H^+,K^+,ATPase$), other actions are secondary to the marked decline of acid secretion. As a result of the reduction of gastric acidity, there is increased secretion of gastrin leading to hypergastrinemia.

396. The answer is a. (*Hardman, p 1579.*) Pregnant women should not take more than a 25% increase in the normal dietary intake of vitamin A, because it is definitely teratogenic, especially in the first trimester of pregnancy. Great caution is to be taken in premenopausal females in the therapy of acne and skin wrinkling in which tretinoin or isotretinoin is the therapeutic agent. None of the other vitamins is particularly teratogenic, except perhaps vitamin D.

397. The answer is c. (*Hardman, pp 1578–1579, 1533.*) Fat-soluble vitamins, especially vitamins A and D, can be stored in massive amounts and, hence, have a potential for serious toxicities. Water-soluble vitamins are easily excreted by the kidney and toxic accumulation rarely occurs.

398. The answer is a. (*Hardman, pp 1547–1542.*) The NRC has a Food and Nutrition Board, which has the function of selecting the levels of vitamins, minerals, and other substances that are necessary to achieve maximum nutritional health. The levels are reviewed periodically and determined by study of the nutritional needs of healthy persons. The FDA is responsible for the labeling of nutritional products, but it does not determine the RDAs.

399. The answer is e. *(Hardman, p 1563.)* The toxicity of INH is mainly on the peripheral and central nervous systems (PNS, CNS). This is attributable to competition of INH with pyridoxal phosphate for apotryptophanase. This results in a relative deficiency of pyridoxine, which causes peripheral neuritis, insomnia, and muscle twitching among other effects.

400. The answer is c. *(Hardman, p 924.)* Dioctyl sodium sulfosuccinate (docusate) is a detergent that, when given orally, softens the stool and prevents straining. Mineral oil also softens the stool, but it tends to inhibit the absorption of fat-soluble vitamins and other nutrients. Castor oil, phenolphthalein, and cascara sagrada are strong laxatives and cause watery stools.

401. The answer is d. *(Hardman, p 913.)* Sucralfate is a sulfated disaccharide that contains polyaluminum hydroxide. It has primarily protective properties and attaches firmly to ulcer craters. It has no significant acid-neutralizing properties.

402–403. The answers are 402-g, 403-a. *(Hardman, pp 1529–1532, 1582–1585.)* Calcitriol (1,25-dihydroxyvitamin D) is the most active form of vitamin D. It is formed by the kidney. When the Ca blood level rises, the kidney produces 24,25-dihydroxyvitamin D, a much less active form. Vitamin D can be manufactured in the body by the action of sunlight on the skin. Its main action is to increase Ca absorption in the gut. Thus, vitamin D subserves important hormonal functions in Ca homeostasis.

Levodopa is converted to dopamine in the peripheral tissues by dopa decarboxylase, which has pyridoxine as a cofactor. Excess of this vitamin will increase this reaction, which is an undesirable effect because dopamine does not cross the blood-brain barrier where the therapeutic effect is desired.

404–405. The answers are 404-e, 405-c. *(Hardman, pp 1555–1557, 1559–1561.)* Angular stomatitis, dermatitis, and corneal vascularization are considered classic signs of human riboflavin deficiency, although multiple B vitamins may be involved.

The classic therapy of the bizarre CNS signs and symptoms of withdrawal in severe alcoholics (Wernicke's syndrome) is intravenous administration of thiamine plus glucose infusion. Alcoholics generally have other deficiencies of vitamins, especially riboflavin and niacin.

406–407. The answers are 406-c, 407-g. (*Hardman, pp 907–909, 926–927.*) Omeprazole, which is an inhibitor of the parietal cell $H^+,K^+,ATPase$ pump (proton pump), is the most effective means of decreasing gastric acidity. This makes it the ideal agent to treat Zollinger-Ellison syndrome, which results from increased gastric secretion due to gastrinomas.

Loperamide is an opiate that is poorly absorbed from the GI tract but still retains the ability to inhibit peristalsis. It is useful in diarrheas that are just symptomatic and are not due to infection or organic pathology, such as inflammatory bowel disease.

408–409. The answers are 408-e, 409-c. (*Hardman, pp 922–923.*) Lactulose is a disaccharide that is not absorbed and, thus, acts as an osmotic agent in the gut. In the colon, lactulose is broken down by bacteria to lactic, formic, and acetic acids plus carbon dioxide, which tend to also increase motility.

Phenolphthalein, like anthraquinones and other irritant phenolic compounds, is a stimulant laxative. Colonic peristalsis is increased by stimulation of sensory nerve endings in the mucosa of the intestine. Phenolphthalein also enhances entrance of water and salts into the bowel.

410–411. The answers are 410-i, 411-d. (*Hardman, pp 156, 622, 624.*) Misoprostol, a methyl analogue of PGE_1, is used in the prevention of ulcers that are caused by NSAIDs, especially in patients with rheumatoid arthritis. Misoprostol inhibits gastric secretion. Because of its stimulatory effect on the uterus, it is contraindicated in women of childbearing age. Prostaglandins, especially PGE_2 and PGI_2, stimulate inhibitory G protein, which controls adenylate cyclase, so as to decrease the production of cAMP and, thus, decrease the action of the $H^+,K^+,ATPase$ pump through protein kinase. Aspirin and other NSAIDs inhibit the synthesis of prostaglandins, allowing stimulatory G protein to be activated by other mechanisms and, thus, allowing the parietal cell to secrete more acid.

Endocrine Syst

Anabolic steroids
Corticosteroids
Male sex hormones
Female sex hormones
Oral fertility agents

Hyperglycemics
Insulins
Oral hypoglyce
Parathyroid agents
Thyroid agents

Questions

DIRECTIONS: Each item below contains a question or incomplete statement followed by suggested responses. Select the **one best** response to each question.

412. The mechanism of action of etidronate disodium is most likely related to

a. An unusual form of phosphorus (P)
b. Inhibition of both normal and abnormal bone resorption
c. Hyperphosphatemia
d. Excretion unchanged in the urine
e. Inhibition of the formation of hydroxyapatite crystals

413. Glucocorticoid synthesis is under direct control of the

a. Hypothalamus
b. Posterior pituitary
c. Adrenal medulla
d. Corticotropin-releasing factor (CRF)
e. Adrenocorticotropic hormone (ACTH)

414. A 75-year-old male, postprostatectomy for carcinoma of the prostate with local metastasis found during surgery, would best be treated with which of the following?

a. Mifepristone
b. Spironolactone
c. Aminoglutethimide
d. Leuprolide
e. Fludrocortisone

5. A naturally occurring substance that is useful in treating Paget's disease of the bone is

a. Etidronate
b. Cortisol
— c. Calcitonin
d. Parathyroid hormone (PTH)
e. Thyroxine (T_4)

416. Neutral protamine Hagedorn (NPH) differs from extended insulin Zn suspension in which of the following actions?

a. It activates receptor tyrosine kinases
b. It causes movement of intracellular glucose transporters to the cell membrane
c. Following subcutaneous injection, it reaches peak plasma concentrations in 6 to 10 h
— d. It has a shorter duration of action
e. It increases lipogenesis

417. The preferred thyroid preparation for maintenance replacement therapy is which of the following drugs?

a. Desiccated thyroid
b. Liothyronine
c. Protirelin
— d. Levothyroxine
e. Liotrix

418. A patient becomes markedly tetanic following a recent thyroidectomy. This symptom can be rapidly reversed by the administration of

a. Vitamin D
b. Calcitonin
c. PTH
d. Plicamycin (mithramycin)
— e. Calcium gluconate (CaG)

419. A 75-year-old diabetic female on an oral hypoglycemic agent becomes light-headed and has profuse sweating. A blood glucose is below normal. Which of the following agents is responsible for these findings?

   a. Pioglitazone
   b. Glipizide
   c. Acarbose
   d. Metformin

420. Metyrapone is useful in testing the endocrine functioning of the

   a. α cells of pancreatic islets
   b. β cells of pancreatic islets
   c. Neurohypophysis
   d. Pituitary-adrenal axis
   e. Leydig's cells of the testes

421. Of the following mechanisms of anti-inflammatory and immunosuppressive effects of glucocorticoids, which one is uniformly observed?

   a. Increased influx of leukocytes to the site of inflammation
   b. Reduced formation of lipocortins
   c. Reduced capillary permeability and edema at the inflammatory site
   d. Increased prostaglandin formation
   e. Enhanced formation of interleukins (IL-1, IL-2)

422. Bromocriptine is used to treat some cases of amenorrhea because it

   a. Stimulates release of gonadotropin-releasing hormone (GnRH)
   b. Stimulates the ovary directly
   c. Is an estrogen antagonist that enhances gonadotropin release
   d. Inhibits prolactin release
   e. Increases the synthesis of follicle-stimulating hormone (FSH)

423. Tamoxifen is used to treat some breast cancers because of its ability to

   a. Utilize its androgenic properties in retarding tumor growth
   b. Prevent estrogen synthesis by the ovary
   c. Enhance glucocorticoid treatment
   d. Act as an estrogen antagonist
   e. Act as a potent progestin

424. Concern is raised in an 86-year-old male with non-insulin-dependent diabetes mellitus (NIDDM), or type II diabetes, about the possibility of hypoglycemia when considering the use of an oral hypoglycemic agent. Which of the following antidiabetic drugs is least likely to cause hypoglycemia?

a. Metformin
b. Chlorpropamide
c. Insulin
d. Glyburide

425. The most dangerous adverse reaction to the administration of methimazole is

a. Hypothyroidism
b. Arthralgia
c. Jaundice
d. Agranulocytosis
e. Renal toxicity

426. The initial and crucial event that enables glyburide to cause the pancreatic β cells to release insulin is

a. Increased potassium (K) efflux
b. Binding to receptors on the adenosine triphosphate (ATP)–sensitive K⁺ channels
c. Closing of voltage-dependent Ca channels
d. Decreased phosphorylation reactions
e. Hyperpolarization

427. The treatment of myxedema coma can include which of the following agents?

a. Thyroglobulin
b. Levothyroxine
c. Lithium
d. Propylthiouracil (PTU)
e. Protirelin

428. The "minipill" containing only a progestin, rather than a combination estrogen-progestin oral contraceptive, was developed because progestin alone

a. Results in less depression and cholestatic jaundice
b. Is a more effective contraceptive agent than the two combined
c. Results in a more regular menstrual cycle
d. Is thought to be less likely to induce endometriosis
e. Is thought to be less likely to induce cardiovascular disorders

429. Parathyroid hormone has which one of the following effects?

a. Increased mobilization of Ca from bone
b. Decreased active absorption of Ca from the small intestine
c. Decreased renal tubular reabsorption of Ca
d. Decreased resorption of phosphate from bone
e. Decreased excretion of phosphate

430. A 60-year-old diabetic male is treated with pioglitazone. What is the mechanism of action of pioglitazone?

a. Increased release of endogenous insulin
b. Decreased plasma glucagon levels
c. Increased hepatic gluconeogenesis
d. Increased target tissue sensitivity to insulin
e. Decreased intestinal absorption of glucose

431. A 25-year-old female suspected of having vitamin D–resistant rickets has decreased blood phosphate levels. Aside from high-dose vitamin D and oral phosphate, an alternative therapeutic approach might be the use of which of the following?

a. Estrogen
b. Pamidronate
c. Hydrochlorothiazide
d. Prednisone
e. Calcitrol

432. A 47-year-old premenopausal female with endometriosis is treated with danazol. Which of the following adverse effects is associated with danazol?

   a. Weight loss
   b. Abnormal liver function tests
   c. Thrombocytopenia
   d. Heavy menses
   e. Mood disorder

433. Glucocorticoids are powerful anti-inflammatory agents. Which of the following is *not* an anti-inflammatory mechanism of action of glucocorticoids?

   a. Decreased secretion of proteolytic enzymes
   b. Reduction in the release of cytokines, such as IL-1 and IL-2
   c. Decreased number of circulating neutrophils
   d. Impairment of prostaglandin and leukotriene synthesis

434. A 60-year-old diabetic male on an oral hypoglycemic agent develops abnormal liver function tests. Which of the following agents can cause this finding?

   a. Glyburide
   b. Metformin
   c. Troglitazone
   d. Acarbose

435. A 55-year-old postmenopausal female develops weakness, polyuria, and polydipsia. Nephrocalcinosis is detected by a computed tomography (CT) scan. Her serum creatinine is elevated. Which of the following agents may have caused these adverse effects?

   a. Estrogens
   b. Prednisone
   c. PTU
   d. Etidronate
   e. Vitamin D

436. Of the following, which is not associated with the abuse of anabolic steroids by athletes?

  a. Retention of fluid
  b. Feminization in males
  c. Decreased spermatogenesis
  d. Depression
  e. Anorexia

437. Of the following, which drug does not increase the need for insulin?

  a. Epinephrine
  b. Hydrocortisone
  c. Chlorthalidone
  d. Dexamethasone
  e. Ethanol (acute ingestion)

438. A 60-year-old male develops elevation of blood pressure, hyperglycemia, decreased bone density, and occult blood in his stool. Which of the following agents is associated with these adverse effects?

  a. Hydrochlorothiazide
  b. Pamidronate
  c. Finasteride
  d. Prednisone
  e. Metformin

439. A 40-year-old male with a symmetrically enlarged thyroid gland associated with elevated levels of T_3 and T_4 is treated with PTU. What is the principal mechanism of action of PTU?

  a. Iodide transport into the cell
  b. Release of T_4 and T_3 to the blood
  c. Inhibition of thyroidal peroxidase
  d. Inhibition of proteolysis of thyroglobulin
  e. Inhibition of iodination and coupling of thyroglobulin

440. Which of the following adverse reactions is *not* associated with the administration of chlorpropamide?

  a. Water retention
  b. Increased tolerance to ethanol
  c. Hypoglycemia
  d. Hyponatremia

441. A 40-year-old male suspected of having adrenal insufficiency is treated with a synthetic derivative of cosyntropin to assess adrenocortical activity. Which of the following enzymes is activated by cosyntropin?

  a. Adenyl cyclase
  b. Mitogen-activated protein kinase
  c. Phosphoinositol 3-kinase
  d. Acetylcholinesterase (AChE)
  e. Phospholipase C
  f. Cyclic guanosine 5'-monophosphate (cGMP) phosphodiesterase

442. A 60-year-old male alcoholic treated for type II diabetes mellitus develops lactic acidosis. Which of the following oral hypoglycemic agents might cause this adverse effect?

  a. Glyburide
  b. Metformin
  c. Acarbose
  d. Rosiglitazone
  e. Chlorpropamide

443. A 25-year-old male with hypogonadism is treated with a synthetic androgen. Which of the following is activated by a synthetic androgen?

  a. Tyrosine kinase receptors
  b. G protein–coupled receptors
  c. Heat shock protein–bound receptors
  d. Muscarinic receptors
  e. Cytokine receptors

444. A drug-drug interaction is possible with sildenafil and which of the following agents?

a. Dobutamide
b. Alprostadil
c. Digoxin
d. Atenolol
e. Nitrates

445. Which of the following drugs is least likely to cause hyperglycemia and hypokalemia?

a. Hydrocortisone
b. Chlorpropamide
c. Hydrochlorothiazide
d. Furosemide
e. Prednisone

446. A 40-year-old nulliparous female having difficulty with becoming pregnant is treated with clomiphene. How would clomiphene be classified?

a. An estrogen
b. An antiestrogen
c. A progestin
d. An antiprogestin

447. A 22-year-old female who requests a postcoital contraceptive after being raped would best be treated with which of the following?

a. Mifepristone
b. Spironolactone
c. Aminoglutethimide
d. Leuprolide
e. Fludrocortisone

448. A 65-year-old diabetic male with erectile dysfunction would be best treated with which of the following?

a. Sildenafil
b. Gossypol
c. Androstenedione
d. Finasteride
e. Calcitonin

449. A 35-year-old male with primary adrenal insufficiency would best be treated with which of the following?

a. Mifepristone
b. Methandrostenolone
c. Misoprostol
d. Leuprolide
e. Fludrocortisone

DIRECTIONS: Each group of questions below consists of lettered options followed by a set of numbered items. For each numbered item, select the **one** lettered option with which it is **most** closely associated. Each lettered option may be used once, more than once, or not at all.

Questions 450–452

For each inhibitory effect on the synthesis of thyroid hormone listed below, select the agent that causes it.

a. Potassium perchlorate
b. Methimazole
c. Triiodothyronine
d. ^{131}I
e. I^-

450. Inhibits, by acting as a competitor, the accumulation of I^- in thyroid follicular cells

451. Inhibits the peroxidase-catalyzed oxidation of I^- and, thus, interferes with the incorporation of I^- into an organic structure

452. Inhibits the peroxidase-catalyzed coupling of iodotyrosines to form iodothyronines

453. A 53-year-old female with NIDDM is started on a sulfonylurea. Which of the following is one mechanism of action of sulfonylureas?

  a. They increase insulin synthesis
  b. They release preformed insulin
  c. They directly promote glucose uptake by muscle, liver, and adipose tissue
  d. They decrease insulin resistance

454. A 29-year-old female who takes levothyroxine following her thyroidectomy becomes pregnant. If the dosage is not changed, she will become

  a. Hyperthyroid
  b. Euthyroid
  c. Hypothyroid

455. A 37-year-old female with Graves' disease who requires antithyroid therapy becomes pregnant. Which antithyroid drug is safest?

  a. Potassium iodide (KI)
  b. Methimazole
  c. PTU
  d. Potassium perchlorate ($KClO_4$)

Questions 456–458

Match each statement with the correct drug.

  a. Aldosterone
  b. Clomiphene
  c. Fludrocortisone
  d. Isophane insulin (NPH)
  e. Methimazole
  f. Ethinyl estradiol
  g. PTU
  h. Salicylates
  i. Spironolactone
  j. Tamoxifen

456. This drug promotes the synthesis of factors II, VII, IX, and X and may interfere with the effect of warfarin or may result in thromboembolic phenomena

d **457.** The therapeutic effect of this drug is reduced by glucocorticoids, epinephrine, hydrochlorothiazide, and levothyroxine.

i **458.** This drug reduces the growth of facial hair in idiopathic hirsutism or hirsutism that is secondary to androgen excess

459. A 36-year-old male has had a thyroidectomy and now requires maintenance therapy. Which of the following is the drug of choice?

  a. KI
  b. PTU
  c. Triiodothyronine
  d. T_4

460. A 27-year-old female is diagnosed with hypercortisolism. To determine whether cortisol production is independent of the pituitary gland, you decide to suppress ACTH production by giving a high-potency glucocorticoid. Which glucocorticoid is the best for this indication?

  a. Triamcinolone
  b. Prednisone
  c. Hydrocortisone
  d. Dexamethasone
  e. Methylprednisolone

461. A 22-year-old female carrying a preterm pregnancy (33 weeks) is in labor. Which of the following drugs can be given to the mother to promote fetal lung maturity?

  a. Betamethasone
  b. Fludrocortisone
  c. Metyrapone
  d. Spironolactone
  e. Triamcinolone

462. A 48-year-old female is diagnosed with small-cell lung carcinoma with ectopic production of ACTH. An adrenocortical antagonist (drug X) is given, and cortisol levels decrease significantly. Following treatment, the patient complains of excess hair growth and swelling of the legs. What is drug X?

- a. Metyrapone
- b. Aminoglutethimide
- c. Spironolactone
- d. Ketoconazole

463. A 22-year-old male with a five-year history of bronchial asthma has developed increased frequency and severity of acute asthmatic attacks. A low dose of which inhaled steroid could be added to his treatment regimen?

- a. Prednisolone
- b. Amcinonide
- c. Beclomethasone
- d. Cortisone
- e. Fluocinolone

464. A 76-year-old male complains of progressive difficulty starting his stream on urinating and having to get up at least once each night to urinate. Rectal examination reveals a generally enlarged, smooth-surfaced prostate. Prostatic serum antigen is 0.2 nanograms per milliliter (ng/mL). Finasteride therapy is begun and results in improved urine flow and decreased prostate size. What is this drug's mechanism of action?

- a. Inhibition of the testosterone receptor
- b. Inhibition of steroid 5α-reductase
- c. Inhibition of testosterone synthesis
- d. Inhibition of the GnRH receptor

Questions 465–467

For each patient, select the drug that was given.

a. Spironolactone
b. Furosemide
c. Clomiphene
d. Propranolol
e. Medroxyprogesterone
f. Chlorpropamide
g. Plicamycin
h. Phentolamine

465. A 25-year-old female complains of increasing anxiety and restlessness. Physical examination reveals tachycardia and tremors. Palpation of the neck reveals a 3-cm nodule on her thyroid gland. While awaiting laboratory confirmation of the diagnosis, she is given a drug that diminishes her tachycardia and tremors.

466. A 48-year-old male with a three-year history of carcinoma of the colon complains of intense pain in his hips. X-rays suggest tumor infiltrates. His serum Ca is 11.5 milliequivalents per liter (mEq/L). A therapeutic regimen is begun that contains a drug that lowers the serum Ca to 8.9 mEq/L.

467. A 50-year-old female had a radical mastectomy three years ago for hormone-dependent breast adenocarcinoma. She is now complaining of shortness of breath, and chest X-ray shows diffuse lung metastases. As part of her therapeutic regimen, she is given intramuscular hormone replacement therapy (HRT).

468. A patient with no history of prior disease and taking sildenafil might develop which of the following adverse effects?

a. Acute pulmonary edema
b. Severe headaches
c. Amylasemia
d. Priapism
e. Profuse sweating

Endocrine System

Answers

412. The answer is e. *(Hardman, pp 1537–1538.)* Etidronate is used in the treatment of Paget's disease of bone. The compound is classified as a diphosphonate. It can be administered orally or by injection. The drug affects both normal and abnormal bone resorption and appears to reduce the activity of osteoclasts and osteoblasts. It inhibits the formation, growth, and dissolution of hydroxyapatite crystals, which is probably its main mechanism of action. There occurs a significant reduction in serum Ca following several days of intravenous therapy with etidronate. The drug has a half-life of about 6 h and is excreted unchanged in the urine. Etidronate has also been used to treat patients with hypercalcemia that may be associated with various neoplastic diseases.

413. The answer is e. *(Hardman, pp 1461–1464.)* Glucocorticoid synthesis is under the control of ACTH. In response to the release of CRF, corticotropin is elaborated from the anterior pituitary gland. It is a polypeptide of 39 amino acids. In the body, cortisol (hydrocortisone) exerts a negative feedback mechanism to suppress the release of corticotropin. Corticotropin affects lipid metabolism by producing a stimulatory effect on lipolysis, which results in an elevated plasma concentration of free fatty acids. The drug is used in the diagnosis of adrenal insufficiency (e.g., primary adrenal insufficiency). When it is given intravenously, its half-life is short, lasting about 15 min. A synthetic form of corticotropin is cosyntropin, which contains only the first 24 amino acids of the peptide.

414. The answer is d. *(Katzung, pp 704, 942.)* Leuprolide is a peptide that is related to GnRH or luteinizing hormone–releasing hormone (LHRH). This agent is used to treat metastatic prostate carcinoma. A hypogonadal state is produced in the patient from the continuous administration of leuprolide, by its capacity to inhibit gonadotropin release. Testosterone levels in the body become significantly reduced.

415. The answer is c. *(Hardman, pp 1536–1537.)* Calcitonin is useful in the therapy of Paget's disease of bone (osteitis deformans). Calcitonin therapy reduces urinary hydroxyproline excretion and serum alkaline phosphatase activity and provides some symptomatic relief. Presumably, these effects result from the ability of calcitonin to inhibit bone resorption. Side effects of long-term therapy with this hormone can include nausea, edema of the hands, and urticaria. The appearance of neutralizing antibodies may explain the development of resistance to treatment. Etidronate is a synthetic drug that is useful in Paget's disease. The compound is orally effective and lacks the antigenicity associated with calcitonin.

416. The answer is d. (*Hardman, pp 1491–1493, 1500–1501.*) Neutral protamine Hagedorn is obtained from animal sources (beef and pork) and by recombinant deoxyribonucleic acid (DNA) techniques to yield human insulin. Protamine and Zn are contained in NPH insulin. Following subcutaneous injection, it has a maximum effect of 8 to 10 h that corresponds to its peak plasma concentrations (6 to 10 h). The duration of action is 18 to 26 h, which is shorter than the duration of action of extended insulin Zn suspension. On the cellular membrane, insulin binds to receptor tyrosine kinases. The activation of these receptor tyrosine kinases leads to phosphorylation reactions and the movement of glucose transporters from the intracellular space to the membranes, where they facilitate the entrance of glucose into the cell. Insulin lowers plasma glucose levels, increases lipogenesis, decreases lipolysis and ketogenesis, and enhances the uptake of amino acids to promote protein synthesis and growth of tissues.

417. The answer is d. (*Katzung, pp 648–615.*) The drug of choice for maintenance replacement therapy of hypothyroidism is levothyroxine (LT_4). Monitoring of plasma blood levels of T_3 and T_4 from the administration of LT_4 causes less difficulty than the monitoring of plasma hormone levels from liothyronine (T_3) because considerable fluctuation can occur with plasma concentrations of T_3. In addition, T_3 has a shorter half-life. Liotrix is a mixture of T_4 and T_3 in a ratio of 4:1 that is designed to resemble the physiologic secretion of the thyroid gland. When liotrix is administered, the T_4 component is converted to T_3 in the body, and T_3, therefore, is actually not needed. It does not appear that liotrix provides any therapeutic advantage over LT_4 by itself for the usual treatment of hypothyroidism. The treatment of hypothyroidism with desiccated thyroid is obsolete. Protirelin, a synthetic tripeptide, is chemically identical to thyrotropin-releasing hormone (TRH). This compound is used for the diagnosis of mild cases of hypothyroidism or hyperthyroidism.

418. The answer is e. *(Hardman, p 1523.)* Administration of intravenous CaG would immediately correct the tetany that might occur in a patient in whom a thyroidectomy was recently performed. Parathyroid hormone would act more slowly but could be given for its future stabilizing effect. Long-term control of a patient after a thyroidectomy can be obtained with vitamin D and dietary therapy. Calcitonin is a hypocalcemic antagonist of parathyroid hormone. Plicamycin (mithramycin) is used to treat Paget's disease and hypercalcemia. The dose employed is about one-tenth the amount used for plicamycin's cytotoxic action.

419. The answer is b. *(Katzung, pp 726–727.)* Glipizide is a second-generation oral hypoglycemic classified as a sulfonylurea. It causes the release of insulin from the β cells of the pancreas. Because of its shorter half-life than glyburide, it is less likely to cause hypoglycemia. Glipizide is contraindicated in patients with liver disease because it is metabolized in the liver. Care should be taken in the elderly because of their propensity to develop hypoglycemia, which is perhaps due to decreased hepatic and renal function that is evident in this patient population. Metformin, acarbose, and pioglitazone do not produce serious hypoglycemic reactions.

420. The answer is d. *(Hardman, pp 1482–1483.)* Metyrapone, because it decreases serum levels of cortisol by inhibiting the 11β-hydroxylation of steroids in the adrenal, can be used to assess the function of the pituitary-adrenal axis. When metyrapone is administered orally or intravenously to normal persons, the adrenohypophysis will secrete an increased amount of ACTH. This will cause a normal adrenal gland to synthesize increased amounts of 17-hydroxylated steroids that can be measured in the urine. However, patients who have disease of the hypothalamico-pituitary complex are not able to respond to administration of metyrapone by producing increased amounts of ACTH; consequently, no increased levels of 17-hydroxylated steroids would be detected in the urine. Before administering the drug, the ability of the adrenal gland to respond to ACTH must be tested.

421. The answer is c. *(Hardman, pp 1470–1472.)* Glucocorticoid compounds are used in therapy because of their anti-inflammatory and immunosuppressive properties. These steroids prevent the movement of neutrophils from the blood to the site of inflammation and cause a redistribution of leukocytes, which also reduces their influx to the site of inflammation.

Glucocorticoids decrease the synthesis of prostaglandins by causing the production of lipocortin, which inhibits the enzyme phospholipase A2. With the inhibition of phospholipase A2, arachidonic acid is not released and, as a consequence, the synthesis of the prostaglandins is decreased or prevented. Glucocorticoids decrease capillary permeability and edema in the site of inflammation by decreasing vasodilation. These drugs inhibit the effects of IL-1, IL-2, tumor necrosis factor (TNF), macrophage migration inhibitory factor (MIF), and other components of the inflammatory and immune responses.

422. The answer is d. *(Hardman, pp 1371–1372.)* High prolactin levels in the serum result in amenorrhea, for reasons that are not known. Bromocriptine inhibits prolactin secretion through its dopaminergic action. This compound, a semisynthetic ergot derivative, appears to be a dopamine receptor agonist. It is administered orally to the patient and, in most cases, menses occurs after a month of therapy.

423. The answer is d. *(Hardman, pp 1275–1276.)* Tamoxifen is an estrogen antagonist used in the treatment of breast cancer. Postmenopausal women with metastases to soft tissue and whose tumors contain an estrogen receptor are more likely to respond to this agent. Little benefit is derived from tamoxifen if the tumor does not have estrogen receptors.

424. The answer is a. *(Hardman, p 1510.)* Although the mechanism of action of metformin and other biguanides is unclear, biguanides virtually never cause hypoglycemia. They operate independently of pancreatic β cells but are not useful in insulin-dependent diabetes mellitus (IDDM). Some possible mechanisms of action are direct stimulation of glycolysis in peripheral tissues, increased sensitivity to insulin, and reduction of glucagon levels.

425. The answer is d. *(Hardman, pp 1398–1400.)* Methimazole is classified as a thioamide and is used in the treatment of hyperthyroidism. It prevents the organification of I⁻ by blocking the oxidation of I⁻ to active I and also inhibits coupling of iodotyrosines. Excessive treatment with this drug may induce hypothyroidism. Some other adverse reactions reported for methimazole include skin rash, fever, jaundice, nephritis, arthralgia, and edema. Agranulocytosis, which is a very serious reaction and may be fatal, is the most dangerous adverse reaction, but it occurs in less than 1% of patients. Patients should be carefully monitored while they are taking this medication because agranulocytosis appears without warning.

426. The answer is b. *(Hardman, pp 1507–1510.)* Glyburide is an oral hypoglycemic agent that is classified as a sulfonylurea derivative. This compound is used in the treatment of NIDDM. For hypoglycemic action, glyburide needs functional β cells in the pancreas, because it is ineffective in depancreatized or severely insulin-deficient patients. Sulfonylurea compounds stimulate the release of insulin from the pancreas by a proposed mechanism of action involving the initial binding of the drug to a receptor on the ATP-sensitive K channels in the cell. As a consequence of this drug-receptor interaction, there is an inhibition of K efflux from the cell, which then produces depolarization of the membrane. The depolarization of the membrane opens voltage-dependent Ca channels to allow the entrance of Ca into the cell. The increased Ca concentration stimulates phosphorylation reactions, followed by the process of exocytosis, which causes the release of insulin from the β cells. Other drugs, such as diazoxide and epinephrine, reduce insulin secretion by causing hyperpolarization of the cell, decreasing Ca ion influx, and thereby preventing the process of exocytosis for the release of insulin.

427. The answer is b. *(Hardman, 1396.)* Myxedema coma is a medical emergency and should be treated as soon as the diagnosis is established. Treatment involves the use of several drugs to correct this condition. It appears that the selection of either LT$_4$, liothyronine, or liotrix is appropriate. LT$_4$, however, is the drug of choice. Supportive treatment of symptoms is also indicated. Maintenance of respiration and administration of fluids and electrolytes, along with glucose if hypoglycemia is diagnosed, should be provided. Because adrenal insufficiency may be present, administration of glucocorticoids is initially recommended.

Thyroglobulin, a protein of high molecular weight, is a component of the thyroid gland. Although preparations are available, this drug is not indicated in myxedema coma. Protirelin is a synthetic thyrotropin-stimulating hormone that is used in the diagnosis of thyroid function. Although lithium was once tested as a drug to treat hyperthyroidism because it induced hypothyroidism, lithium has no place in the therapy of hyperthyroidism. In addition, PTU is an antithyroid drug used in the management of hyperthyroidism.

428. The answer is e. *(Hardman, pp 1432, 1434.)* The combination of estrogen and progestin is a more effective means of contraception than is progestin alone. Menstruation will occur with progestin alone, but it may be irregular. Estrogen is thought to cause the increased incidence of thrombophlebitis and cerebral and coronary thromboses that are found in women taking combined oral contraceptives.

429. The answer is a. *(Hardman, pp 1525–1528.)* Parathyroid hormone is synthesized by and released from the parathyroid gland; increased synthesis of PTH is a response to low serum Ca concentrations. Resorption and mobilization of Ca and phosphate from bone are increased in response to elevated PTH concentrations. Replacement of body stores of Ca is enhanced by the capacity of PTH to promote increased absorption of Ca by the small intestine in concert with vitamin D, which is the primary factor that enhances intestinal Ca absorption. Parathyroid hormone also causes an increased renal tubular reabsorption of Ca and excretion of phosphate. As a consequence of these effects, the extracellular Ca concentration becomes elevated.

430. The answer is d. *(Hardman, p 1510.)* Pioglitazone is a thiazolidinedione whose mechanism of action is dependent on the presence of insulin. It reduces plasma glucose, insulin, and lipid concentrations. It appears to increase target tissue sensitivity to insulin by binding as a highly selective agonist to peroxisome proliferator–activated receptors that regulate the transcription of insulin-responsive genes involved in control of glucose and lipid metabolism. One of the outcomes is an increase in the number of glucose transporters.

431. The answer is e. *(Katzung, pp 744, 748.)* Vitamin D_3 is hydroxylated to 25-OHD$_3$ (calcifediol). Calcifediol is then hydroxylated in the kidney to the most active form of vitamin D, which is 1,25-dihydroxyvitamin D (calcitriol). Calcitriol has a rapid onset of action and a short half-life. The administration of calcitriol causes the elevation of serum Ca levels by enhancing the intestinal absorption of Ca. Calcitriol is indicated in vitamin D deficiency, particularly in patients with chronic renal failure or renal tubular disease, hypoparathyroidism, osteomalacia, and rickets. Serum phosphate levels usually increase with prolonged treatment.

432. The answer is b. *(Katzung, pp 698–699.)* Danazol is a 17α-ethinyl testosterone derivative used to treat endometriosis. It appears to be more effective than an estrogen-progestin combination. Because danazol is an androgen derivative, some of the adverse reactions include liver dysfunction, virilism (acne, hirsutism, oily skin, reduced breast size), and reduction in high-density lipoprotein (HDL) cholesterol levels. Other adverse reactions reported for danazol are amenorrhea, weight gain, sweating, vasomotor flushing, and edema. When danazol therapy for endometriosis was compared with the estrogen-progestin regimen, few women discontinued the treatment with danazol because of adverse reactions.

433. The answer is c. *(Hardman, p 1471. Katzung, p 665.)* Glucocorticoids actually increase the number of circulating neutrophils as inhibition of margination and migration occurs. Paradoxically, this is an anti-inflammatory effect as neutrophils had not been reaching the sites where they were needed. All of the other choices are anti-inflammatory mechanisms of glucocorticoid action.

434. The answer is c. *(Katzung, p 729.)* Hepatic dysfunction has occurred particularly with the use of troglitazone, necessitating its removal from the market. Patients treated with other thiazolidinediones should be monitored for this possibility.

435. The answer is e. *(Hardman, p 1533.)* Enthusiastic overmedication with vitamin D may lead to a toxic syndrome called *hypervitaminosis D*. The initial symptoms can include weakness, nausea, weight loss, anemia, and mild acidosis. As the excessive doses are continued, signs of nephrotoxicity are manifested, such as polyuria, polydipsia, azotemia, and eventually nephrocalcinosis. In adults, osteoporosis can occur. Also, there is CNS impairment, which can result in mental retardation and convulsions.

436. The answer is e. *(Hardman, pp 1451–1452.)* The use of anabolic steroids by athletes has become quite alarming in recent years. These steroids, which have androgenic and anabolic effects, are used to improve the performance of athletes in various competitive sports. Continued use of anabolic steroids induces mood changes, as well as mental disorders ranging from depression to psychosis. The androgenic properties of these drugs cause masculinization in females and may produce feminization in males. This latter effect is due to increased formation of estrogens. In addition, these steroids decrease production of endogenous testosterone by the testes and may cause a reduction in spermatogenesis. The weight gain that occurs with the administration of anabolic steroids may be due to fluid retention and an improved appetite rather than actual tissue growth. These drugs cause liver damage and increase the risk of cardiovascular diseases.

437. The answer is e. *(Hardman, p 1505.)* The regulation of levels of blood glucose by insulin and the general effectiveness of insulin are altered with the coadministration of other drugs. Epinephrine enhances glycogenolysis and thereby elevates glucose in the plasma. Glucocorticoids (e.g., hydrocortisone and dexamethasone) stimulate gluconeogenesis, reduce the peripheral utilization of glucose, and decrease the sensitivity of tissues to insulin. Chlorthalidone, a thiazide-related diuretic, may induce hyperglycemia by inhibition of the release of insulin and decreased use of glucose by peripheral tissues. In the presence of ethanol, the effect of insulin is enhanced. When ethanol is acutely ingested in sufficient quantities, the drug causes an alteration in carbohydrate metabolism that results in hypoglycemia. The exact mechanism of the hypoglycemic effect of ethanol is not known.

438. The answer is d. *(Hardman, pp 1475–1476.)* The incidence of adverse reactions with administration of prednisone is related to dosage and duration. Psychoses, peptic ulceration with or without hemorrhage (possibly leading to guaiac-positive stools), increased susceptibility to infection, edema, osteoporosis, myopathy, and hypokalemic alkalosis can occur. Other adverse reactions include cataracts, hyperglycemia, arrest of growth in children, and iatrogenic Cushing's syndrome. The glucocorticoids are very effective drugs, but they can be very dangerous if not properly administered to a patient.

439. The answer is c. *(Katzung, pp 651–652.)* Propylthiouracil is a thioamide that interferes with the production of thyroid hormone. Its primary action is prevention of thyroid hormone synthesis by blocking thyroid peroxidase catalysis leading to interference with iodine organification.

It also blocks coupling of iodotyrosines. Deiodination of T_4 to T_3 is inhibited by PTU in the periphery.

440. The answer is b. *(Katzung, p 726. Hardman, p 1509.)* The oral hypoglycemic agent chlorpropamide is a sulfonylurea compound. The drug is used to treat selected patients with non-insulin-dependent diabetes mellitus (NIDDM). Chlorpropamide has a duration of action of 1 to 3 days. The adverse reaction of hypoglycemia appears to be more common with chlorpropamide than with the other sulfonylurea oral hypoglycemic agents. In addition, water retention and hyponatremia can be caused by chlorpropamide. This adverse reaction is due to an interaction between antidiuretic hormone (ADH) and chlorpropamide. In the collecting duct region of the nephron, chlorpropamide may enhance the effect of antidiuretic hormone and facilitate its release from the posterior pituitary gland. It is reported that chlorpropamide decreases the tolerance to ethanol—an interaction exhibited by flushing of the skin, particularly in the facial area. This disulfiram-like effect is attributed to the inhibition of the oxidation of acetaldehyde that is formed from the biotransformation of ethanol.

441. The answer is a. *(Hardman, pp 1460, 1464.)* Cosyntropin is related to adrenocorticotropin. It corresponds to the first 24 amino acids of adrenocorticotropin. Cosyntropin complexes with a plasma membrane receptor that brings about the activation of adenylyl cyclase. Adenylyl cyclase catalyzes the formation of cAMP from ATP. In the cytoplasm, cAMP activates cAMP-dependent protein kinase, which participates in the phosphorylation of specific substrate proteins (e.g., enzymes). The phosphorylated protein eventually induces the particular response on the target cell.

The cellular mechanism of action of hydrocortisone, a glucocorticoid, is also related to proteins but not by the enhancement of cAMP production. Hydrocortisone is transported by simple diffusion across the membrane of the cell into the cytoplasm and binds to a specific receptor. The steroid-receptor complex is activated and enters the nucleus, where it regulates transcription of specific gene sequences into ribonucleic acid (RNA). Eventually, messenger RNA (mRNA) is translated to form specific proteins in the cytoplasm that are involved in the steroid-induced cellular response.

442. The answer is b. *(Katzung, pp 727–728.)* Metformin is contraindicated in patients with type II diabetes in a number of instances, including renal disease, liver disease, chronic cardiopulmonary dysfunction leading to hypoxia, and alcoholism.

443. The answer is c. (*Katzung, pp 662–664.*) A variety of drugs that resemble steroid hormones in their structure can traverse cellular membranes and bind to specific cytoplasmic receptors that bind heat shock proteins. Among these are the synthetic androgens. These agents bind reversibly to the cytoplasmic receptor, causing release of the heat shock proteins, followed by an irreversible activation step. Next, the steroid-receptor complex enters the nucleus of the cell and regulates transcription of specific genes into RNA. Eventually, mRNA is formed and causes the synthesis of specific proteins that mediate the steroid response. The response occurs 30 min to several hours after administration of the drug, because a period of time is required for formation of new proteins in the cell.

444. The answer is e. (*Katzung, p 187.*) Sildenafil is effective in many patients with erectile dysfunction. It increases cGMP by inhibiting phosphodiesterase isoform 5. The potentiation of nitrate action by sildenafil is thought to result from both agents increasing the concentration of nitric oxide, which leads to an increase in cGMP, thereby resulting in hypotension.

445. The answer is b. (*Hardman, pp 1468–1470.*) Chlorpropamide is a hypoglycemic agent used for controlling blood glucose levels in patients who have NIDDM. Dilutional hyponatremia, but not hypokalemia, may occur with the chronic use of chlorpropamide. Hydrocortisone and prednisone induce hyperglycemia by enhancing gluconeogenesis in the liver and periphery. In addition, the steroids also promote the release of glucagon from the cells of the pancreas to eventually increase blood glucose levels. Hydrocortisone possesses significant mineralocorticoid activity in addition to its glucocorticoid effect. The mineralocorticoid action of hydrocortisone alters electrolyte metabolism. Hydrocortisone enhances the retention of Na and water in the body and augments the secretion of K, which can lead to hypokalemia. Prednisone also possesses a degree of mineralocorticoid activity and may produce hypokalemia. Furosemide can cause hypokalemia. In addition, it can cause hyperglycemia by inhibiting the release of insulin from the pancreas.

446. The answer is b. (*Hardman, pp 1424–1425. Katzung, pp 699–700.*) Clomiphene binds the estrogen receptor. It typically acts as a partial antagonist; however, it can exhibit full antagonism or no effect at all. It stimulates ovulation in disorders of ovulation and in amenorrheic patients. In patients who fail to ovulate, it is suggested that clomiphene interferes with the negative feedback of endogenous estrogens, thereby increasing the release of LH and FSH by the pituatary.

447. The answer is a. *(Katzung, pp 697–698.)* Mifepristone is structurally related to norethindrone. This compound is classified as a progesterone antagonist with weak agonistic properties. A single dose can function as an emergency postcoital contraceptive. It also can induce an abortion by causing contraction of the myometrium, which leads to detachment of the embryo. The drug is used in single or multiple doses followed by the administration of a prostaglandin to cause the abortion. Estrogens used alone or in combination with progestins have also proven effective in postcoital contraception.

448. The answer is a. *(Katzung, p 187.)* Sildenafil inhibits the action of phosphodiesterase isoform 5, the major phosphodiesterase in the corpus cavernosum that degrades cGMP. Nitric oxide is released on sexual stimulation. This leads to an increase in cGMP. By inhibiting the enzyme, sildenafil causes the accumulation of cGMP. This results in vascular smooth-muscle dilation, allowing increased blood flow into the penis followed by erection.

449. The answer is e. *(Katzung, p 672. Hardman, pp 1477–1478.)* Fludrocortisone is a synthetic steroid compound that exhibits profound mineralocorticoid activity and some glucocorticoid activity. Electrolyte and water metabolisms are affected by the administration of this compound. Fludrocortisone promotes the reabsorption of Na and the urinary excretion of K and hydrogen ions in the collecting duct of the nephron. The drug is indicated for mineralocorticoid replacement therapy in primary adrenal insufficiency.

450–452. The answers are 450-a, 451-b, 452-b. *(Katzung, p 652. Hardman, pp 1397–1406.)* Agents that can interfere directly or indirectly with the synthesis of thyroid hormone are called *thyroid inhibitors*. Perchlorate, an ionic inhibitor, interferes with the ability of the thyroid to concentrate I⁻ by acting as a competitive inhibitor. It is used in patients with iodide-induced hypothyroidism, such as can occur with the antiarrhythmic agent amiodarone.

Methimazole, together with PTU, is classified as an antithyroid drug that interferes directly with thyroid hormone synthesis. Antithyroid drugs interfere with the oxidation and incorporation of I⁻ into any organic form and inhibit the formation of iodothyronines from the peroxidase-mediated coupling of iodotyrosines. These drugs may act by binding to peroxidase, by interacting with substrates, or by interfering with the production of hydrogen peroxide, which (in addition to oxygen) is a biologic oxidant required for the synthesis of thyroid hormones.

Iodine, most ancient of the therapeutic agents for thyroid disorders, inhibits the secretion of thyroid hormone by retarding both the pinocytosis of colloid and proteolysis. This effect is observed in euthyroid as well as hyperthyroid persons.

Triiodothyronine is not classified as a thyroid inhibitor; it is an amino acid derivative of thyronine and results from the oxidative coupling of monoiodotyrosyl and diiodotyrosyl residues. Iodine 131, the most often used radioisotope of I, is rapidly absorbed by the thyroid and is deposited in follicular colloid. From the site of its deposition, ^{131}I causes fibrosis of the thyroid subsequent to pyknosis and necrosis of the follicular cells.

453. The answer is b. *(Hardman, p 1507. Katzung, pp 723–724.)* Three proposed mechanisms for sulfonylurea action are (1) the release of insulin from pancreatic cells, (2) reduction of serum glucagon levels, and (3) increased binding of insulin to tissue receptors. On binding to a specific receptor that is associated with a K channel in cell membranes, sulfonylureas inhibit K efflux, which causes influx of Ca followed by release of preformed insulin.

454. The answer is c. *(Hardman, pp 1395–1396. Katzung, p 647.)* The bound and the free concentration of T₄ will decrease unless this patient receives more drug. In a normal pregnant woman, the thyroid gland will secrete more T₃ and T₄ until the free levels are back in the normal range. However, after thyroidectomy or in any pregnant woman with hypothyroidism, exogenous thyroid hormone is required to maintain normal free levels. Also, the hypothyroid state must be corrected before administering oral contraceptives because they increase levels of thyroid-binding globulin.

455. The answer is c. *(Hardman, p 1401.)* Propylthiouracil is more strongly protein bound and crosses the placenta to a lesser degree than methimazole and is, therefore, the safest antithyroid drug in pregnancy.

456–458. The answers are 456-f, 457-d, 458-i. (*Hardman, pp 707–709, 1419–1421, 1505.*) Ethinyl estradiol is a synthetic estrogen derivative that is orally effective. It is used in combination with progestins as an oral contraceptive. Ethinyl estradiol is also used alone in various gynecologic disorders such as menopausal symptoms, in breast cancer in selected postmenopausal women, and in prostatic carcinoma. A major adverse reaction with ethinyl estradiol and other estrogens involves the coagulation reaction. Estrogens increase the synthesis of vitamin K–dependent factors II, VII, IX, and X. The effect on the coagulation scheme can alter the prothrombin time of persons who are using oral anticoagulants (e.g., warfarin). In addition, estrogens can increase the incidence of thromboembolic disorders through their procoagulation effect.

In the therapy of diabetes mellitus, the effectiveness of insulin to regulate glucose levels in the body can be reduced by simultaneous administration of other drugs. Glucose levels in the body are elevated by the administration of glucocorticoid (e.g., hydrocortisone), dextrothyroxine, epinephrine, thiazide diuretics (e.g., hydrochlorothiazide), and LT_4. The drug-induced hyperglycemia counteracts the hypoglycemic action of insulin preparations. In addition, any drug that induces hyperglycemia can also reduce the effectiveness of the oral hypoglycemic agents such as tolbutamide, acetohexamide, and glyburide.

Spironolactone is classified as a K-sparing diuretic. Spironolactone is a competitive inhibitor of aldosterone. It has a mild diuretic effect but is generally used with other diuretics such as thiazides or loop diuretics to prevent the development of hypokalemia. The drug is also used in endocrinology in the diagnosis and treatment of hyperaldosteronism. Another therapeutic use of spironolactone is in the treatment of hirsutism in females, whether it is idiopathic or related to excessive androgen secretion. The drug causes a decrease in the rate of growth and the density of facial hair, possibly through inhibition of excessive androgen production and an effect on the hair follicle.

459. The answer is e. (*Hardman, p 1395.*) Thyroid hormone is used for HRT in hypothyroidism. T_4 is the hormone of choice because of its consistent potency and prolonged duration of action.

460. The answer is d. (*Hardman, p 1481.*) Of the glucocorticoids listed, dexamethasone is the most potent. The dexamethasone suppression test has several uses—it allows not only complete suppression of pituitary ACTH production, but also accurate measurement of endogenous corticosteroids such as 17-ketosteroids in the urine. The small amount of dexamethasone present contributes minimally to this measurement.

461. The answer is a. *(Katzung, p 668.)* Fetal lung maturation is normally stimulated by cortisol produced in the fetal adrenal gland. When preterm delivery with inadequate maturation of the lungs is anticipated, large doses of glucocorticoid can be given to the mother to speed up the physiologic process. Betamethasone is the preferred agent because it binds to serum proteins to a lesser extent than cortisol and other glucocorticoids, allowing more steroid to cross the placenta.

462. The answer is a. *(Hardman, pp 1482–1483. Katzung, pp 673–674.)* Metyrapone inhibits 11-hydroxylation of steroid precursors, which prevents formation of cortisone and cortisol. These precursors are then diverted into aldosterone and androgen production pathways, which explains the adverse effects of hirsutism and edema.

463. The answer is c. *(Hardman, p 666.)* Inhalation therapy minimizes systemic effects of steroids. Of the agents above, beclomethasone is the only one delivered by metered-dose inhaler (MDI).

464. The answer is b. *(Hardman, p 1453. Katzung, p 705.)* Finasteride is a competitive inhibitor of the steroid 5-reductase, causing reduction in plasma and prostate dihydrotestosterone. Males with benign prostatic hypertrophy (BPH) that are treated with finasteride are found to have decreased prostate size. A change in symptoms related to urination occurs in about one-third of patients.

465. The answer is d. *(Hardman, p 1401.)* In patients who are suspected of having hyperthyroidism, propranolol can be administered to provide temporary relief of the peripheral manifestations of the disease while the patient is further evaluated. Propranolol suppresses adrenergic symptoms such as tremors and tachycardia; it has no effect on the release of thyroid hormones from the gland.

466. The answer is g. *(Hardman, p 1268.)* Plicamycin (mithramycin) can be used to treat hypercalcemia associated with malignancies. Its mechanism of action involves inhibition of Ca reabsorption from bone, leading to a reduction in serum Ca levels.

467. The answer is e. *(Hardman, p 1274.)* Medroxyprogesterone is used as a second-line hormone therapy for metastatic breast or endometrial carcinoma that was previously treated with surgery and radiation.

468. The answer is d. *(Katzung, p 187.)* Sildenafil is used in cases of erectile dysfunction. Although it is a relatively safe drug, it does produce some troubling adverse effects. Prolonged erection, difficulty with orgasm, abnormal ejaculation, blue-green vision discrimination difficulties, and priapism have occurred with use of sildenafil. Patients on vasodilators and those with underlying cardiovascular disease are at risk for developing serious cardiovascular events.

Toxicology

Air pollutants
Alcohols
Heavy metals
Heavy metal antagonists

Herbicides
Organophosphorus insecticides
Insecticide antidotes
Toxic gases

Questions

DIRECTIONS: Each item below contains a question or incomplete statement followed by suggested responses. Select the **one best** response to each question.

469. Convulsions caused by drug poisoning are most commonly associated with

a. Phenobarbital
b. Diazepam
c. Strychnine
d. Chlorpromazine
e. Phenytoin

470. Alkalinization of the urine with sodium bicarbonate is useful in the treatment of poisoning with

a. Aspirin (acetylsalicylic acid)
b. Amphetamine
c. Morphine
d. Phencyclidine
e. Cocaine

471. Which of the following is an agent useful in the treatment of severe poisoning by organophosphorus insecticides, such as parathion?

a. Ethylenediaminotetraacetic acid (EDTA)
b. Pralidoxime (2-PAM)
c. N-acetyl-L-cysteine
d. Carbachol
e. Diethyldithiocarbamic acid

472. N-acetylbenzoquinoneimine is the hepatotoxic metabolite of which drug?

a. Sulindac
b. Acetaminophen
c. Isoniazid
d. Indomethacin
e. Procainamide

473. Rapid intravenous administration of this drug causes hypocalcemic tetany.

a. Dimercaprol
b. Edetate disodium (Na_2EDTA)
c. Deferoxamine
d. Penicillamine
e. N-acetylcysteine

474. Acute intermittent porphyria is a contraindication of the use of

a. Enflurane
b. Nitrous oxide (N_2O)
c. Ketamine
d. Diazepam
e. Thiopental

475. A 15-year-old male attempts suicide with a liquid that causes intense abdominal pain, skeletal muscle cramps, projectile vomiting, severe diarrhea, and difficulty swallowing. On examination, he is found to be volume depleted and is showing signs of alteration of consciousness. Which of the following may account for these symptoms?

a. Arsenic (As)
b. Cadmium (Cd)
c. Iron (Fe)
d. Lead (Pb)
e. Zinc (Zn)

476. Cadmium poisoning is almost as common as Pb and Hg poisoning. Of the following, which is unlikely to be associated with Cd poisoning?

a. Exposure to fumes causes dyspnea, substernal discomfort, myalgias, headaches, and vomiting
b. Chronic exposure results in severe liver injury
c. The most common long-term toxicity is renal
d. In Japan, a Cd intoxication syndrome is known as *itai-itai* (ouch-ouch) because of back, joint, and bone pain

477. A 3-year-old female ingests a bottle of aspirin by accident. Among the therapeutic interventions, which of the following should be included?

a. Dimercaprol
b. Deferoxamine
c. Penicillamine
d. Na_2EDTA
e. Activated charcoal

478. A 50-year-old male chronic alcoholic ingests methanol. Which of the following findings is associated with acute methanol ingestion?

a. Metabolic alkalosis
b. Delirium tremens
c. An atrioventricular conduction defect
d. Blurred vision
e. Tachypnia

479. Of the following drugs, which would not produce a syndrome of flushing, headache, nausea, vomiting, sweating, hypotension, and confusion after ethanol consumption?

a. Amitriptyline
b. Cefoperazone
c. Tolbutamide
d. Metronidazole
e. Disulfiram

480. A 60-year-old male complains of severe headaches, nausea, dizziness, and a diminution in vision. He has a decrease in oxygen (O_2)-carrying capacity without a change in the P_{O_2} of arterial blood. Which of the following might account for these findings?

a. Sulfur dioxide
b. Ozone
c. Nitrogen dioxide
d. Carbon monoxide (CO)
e. Methane

481. Zinc is an essential element for normal growth and development. However, toxicity can occur from excessive exposure. Of the following, which is not a manifestation of chronic poisoning with zinc?

a. Decreased amylase secretion
b. Thrombocytopenia
c. Anemia
d. Encephalopathy
e. Fever

DIRECTIONS: Each group of questions below consists of lettered options followed by a set of numbered items. For each numbered item, select the **one** lettered option with which it is **most** closely associated. Each lettered option may be used once, more than once, or not at all.

Questions 482–483

Many drugs when given to a pregnant woman produce significant adverse effects on the fetus. For each of the drugs below, match the most likely adverse effect.

a. Vaginal adenocarcinoma
b. Congenital goiter, hypothyroidism
c. Masculinization of female fetus
d. "Gray baby" syndrome
e. Prolonged neonatal hypoglycemia
f. Kernicterus

482. Testosterone

483. Methimazole

Questions 484–485

For each patient, select the drug or agent most likely to cause the toxic effect.

a. Aluminum (Al)
b. Bismuth (Bi)
c. CO
d. Dapsone
e. Methanol
f. Gentamicin
g. Pb
h. Metronidazole
i. Primaquine
j. Ethylene glycol
k. Sulfamethoxazole
l. Sulfasalazine
m. Tetracycline

484. A 49-year-old woman is treated for an *Escherichia coli* urinary tract infection (UTI). During treatment, the woman experiences hemolysis.

485. A 3-year-old boy consumed a liquid from a container in the family garage. He shows central nervous system (CNS) depression, acidosis, suppressed respiration, and oxalate crystals in the urine. Besides supportive and corrective measures, ethanol was administered to the child.

Questions 486–487

Certain drugs carry a risk of fetal abnormalities if administered during pregnancy. Match each abnormality with the correct drug.

a. Penicillamine
b. Diethylstilbestrol
c. Prednisone
d. Chloramphenicol
e. Phenobarbital
f. Disulfiram
g. Ethanol
h. Heroin
i. Metronidazole
j. Chlorambucil

486. Malformations of the genitourinary (GU) tract

487. Cutis laxa

Questions 488–489

Death from acute poisoning usually occurs by mechanisms that involve vital systems such as respiration, circulation, or the CNS. Match each clinical picture with the causative agent.

a. Cocaine
b. CO
c. Strychnine
d. Atropine
e. Phenobarbital
f. Heroin
g. Phencyclidine
h. Aspirin
i. Cyanide (Cn)
j. Lysergic acid diethylamide (LSD)

488. Hallucinations, delirium, and coma along with tachycardia and hypertension; hot, dry skin; urinary retention; and dilated pupils

489. Tinnitus, confusion, lethargy, and seizures; hyperventilation and an anion-gap metabolic acidosis

490. A 2-year-old male ingests iron pills by accident. He develops severe abdominal pain and bloody vomitus. Which of the following might be administered to this patient?

a. Dimercaprol
b. Deferoxamine
c. Penicillamine
d. Na$_2$EDTA
e. Activated charcoal

Toxicology

Answers

469. The answer is c. *(Hardman, pp 89–90.)* Strychnine acts as a competitive antagonist of glycine, the predominant postsynaptic inhibitory transmitter in the brain and spinal cord. The fatal adult dose is 50 to 100 mg. Persons poisoned by strychnine suffer convulsions that progress to full tetanic convulsions. Because the diaphragm and thoracic muscles are fully contracted, the patient cannot breathe. Hypoxia eventually causes medullary paralysis and death. Control of the convulsions and respiratory support are the immediate objectives of therapy. Diazepam may be preferred to a barbiturate in controlling the convulsions because it offers less concomitant respiratory depression. Poisoning caused by the other drugs listed in the question is not associated with convulsions but with depression of the CNS.

470. The answer is a. *(Hardman, pp 16–20.)* Sodium bicarbonate is excreted principally in the urine and alkalinizes it. Increasing urinary pH interferes with the passive renal tubular reabsorption of organic acids (such as aspirin and phenobarbital) by increasing the ionic form of the drug in the tubular filtrate. This would increase their excretion. Excretion of organic bases (such as amphetamine, cocaine, phencyclidine, and morphine) would be enhanced by acidifying the urine.

471. The answer is b. *(Hardman, p 170.)* The organophosphorus insecticides inactivate cholinesterases, which results in accumulation of endogenous acetylcholine (ACh) in nerve tissue and effector organs. Very severe cases of acute poisoning should be treated first with atropine followed immediately by intravenous 2-PAM. Atropine inhibits the actions of ACh at muscarinic cholinergic receptors, whereas 2-PAM reactivates the inactivated cholinesterases. The effectiveness of 2-PAM in reversing cholinesterase inhibition depends on early treatment inasmuch as the "aged" inhibited enzyme cannot be reactivated. Diethyldithiocarbamic acid is the active biotransformation product of disulfiram, which is an irreversible inhibitor of aldehyde dehydrogenase. N-acetyl-L-cysteine is an antidote used in the treatment of acetaminophen overdosage to prevent hepatotoxicities. Carbachol is a cholinomimetic drug, and EDTA is a chelating agent. These compounds have no therapeutic value in the treatment of organophosphate poisoning.

472. The answer is b. *(Hardman, pp 632–633.)* Hepatic necrosis can occur with overdosage of acetaminophen. The hepatic toxicity is the result of the biotransformation of acetaminophen to N-acetylbenzoquinoneimine, which reacts with hepatic proteins and glutathione. This metabolite depletes glutathione, stores and produces necrosis. The administration of N-acetyl-L-cysteine restores hepatic concentrations of glutathione and reduces the potential hepatotoxicity. Sulindac is biotransformed to sulindac sulfide, the active form of the drug. Both sulindac and its metabolites are excreted in the urine and in the feces. Indomethacin undergoes a demethylation reaction and an N-deacylation reaction. The parent compound and its metabolites are mainly excreted in the urine. Procainamide is converted to an active metabolite by an acetylation reaction. The product that is formed is N-acetylprocainamide (NAPA). In addition, procainamide is hydrolyzed by amidases. An N-acetylation reaction occurs also in the biotransformation of isoniazid. In the liver, the enzyme N-acetyltransferase converts isoniazid to acetylisoniazid.

473. The answer is b. *(Hardman, pp 1664–1669.)* The chelation agent, Na_2EDTA, causes hypocalcemic tetany on rapid intravenous administration. This effect of Na_2EDTA is not observed on slow infusion (15 mg/min) because extracirculatory stores are available to prevent a significant reduction in plasma Ca levels. When $CaNa_2EDTA$ is given intravenously, hypocalcemia does not develop, even when large doses are required. $CaNa_2EDTA$ is used in the diagnosis and treatment of Pb intoxication. Na_2EDTA is used to treat acute hypercalcemia. The other drugs listed do not cause hypocalcemia. Dimercaprol [British antilewisite (BAL)] forms chelation complexes between its sulfhydryl groups and metals and is used in the treatment of arsenic and Hg poisoning, as well as in certain cases of Pb poisoning in children. Penicillamine is the drug of choice in treating Wilson's disease. The agent is also used in the therapy of Cu, Hg, and Pb poisoning. N-acetyl-L-cysteine is an antidote used in the treatment of overdosage with acetaminophen to prevent hepatotoxicity.

474. The answer is e. *(Hardman, p 323.)* Induction of anesthesia by parenteral administration of thiopental sodium and other barbiturates is absolutely contraindicated in patients who have acute intermittent porphyria. These patients have a defect in regulation of δ-aminolevulinic acid synthetase; thus, administration of a barbiturate that increases this enzyme may cause a dangerous increase in levels of porphyrins. Administration of a barbiturate would exacerbate the symptoms of gastrointestinal and neurologic disturbances, cause extensive demyelination of peripheral and cranial nerves, and could lead to death.

475. The answer is a. *(Hardman, pp 1660–1661.)* Arsenic is an active constituent of fungicides, herbicides, and pesticides. Symptoms of acute toxicity include tightness in the throat, difficulty in swallowing, and stomach pains. Projectile vomiting and severe diarrhea can lead to hypovolemic shock and death. Chronic poisoning may cause peripheral neuritis, anemia, skin keratosis, and capillary dilation leading to hypotension. Dimercaprol is the primary agent used in the treatment of arsenic poisoning.

476. The answer is b. *(Hardman, pp 1663–1664.)* The liver appears to be spared in Cd intoxication. Not so the kidney, which, in chronic exposure, develops proteinuria with extensive damage to the proximal tubule. The symptoms of acute exposure to Cd fumes are substernal discomfort, myalgias, headache, fatigue, and vomiting. These may be followed in severe cases by wheezing, hemoptysis, and pulmonary edema. In certain parts of Japan, where Cd industrial waste is common, a syndrome of osteomalacia and bone deformities accompanied by pain and waddling gait is known as *itai-itai* (ouch-ouch).

477. The answer is e. *(Hardman, p 72.)* Activated charcoal, a fine, black powder with a high adsorptive capacity, is considered to be a highly valuable agent in the treatment of many kinds of drug poisoning. Drugs that are well adsorbed by activated charcoal include primaquine, propoxyphene, dextroamphetamine, chlorpheniramine, phenobarbital, carbamazepine, digoxin, and aspirin. Mineral acids, alkalines, tolbutamide, and other drugs that are insoluble in acidic aqueous solution are not well adsorbed. Charcoal also does not bind Ca, lithium (Li), or Fe.

478. The answer is d. *(Hardman, pp 1681–1682. Katzung, pp 392–393.)* Acute intoxication with methanol is common in chronic alcoholics. Headache, vertigo, vomiting, abdominal pain, dyspnea, blurred vision, and hyperemia of the optic disc can occur. Visual disturbances are caused by damage to retinal cells and the optic nerve by methanol metabolites. Severe cases of intoxication can lead to blindness. Other symptoms include bradycardia, prolonged coma, seizures, acidosis, and death by respiratory depression. Because methanol is biotransformed by alcohol and aldehyde dehydrogenase to highly toxic products (formaldehyde and formic acid, respectively), ethanol, which has a high affinity for the enzyme, is useful in therapy because it reduces the biotransformation of methanol. Other treatments include hemodialysis to enhance removal of methanol and its products and alkalinization to reverse metabolic acidosis. 4-methylprazole, an inhibitor of alcohol dehydrogenase, has also been proposed for treatment. Treatment with ascorbic acid would aggravate the acidosis.

479. The answer is a. *(Hardman, pp 391–392.)* Disulfiram is a pharmacologic adjunct in the treatment of alcoholism. When given to a person who has consumed ethanol, it produces flushing, headache, nausea, vomiting, sweating, hypotension, and confusion. The mechanism involves inhibition of aldehyde dehydrogenase; thus, acetaldehyde accumulates as a result of ethanol metabolism. Many other agents produce disulfiram-like reactions when administered with ethanol: these include cephalosporins (cefoperazine, cefoperazone), phentolamine, metronidazole, and the sulfonylureas (tolbutamide). The tricyclic antidepressant amitriptyline causes sedation. The interaction between ethanol and amitriptyline produces an enhancement of the central depressant properties of ethanol.

480. The answer is d. *(Hardman, pp 1676–1678. Katzung, pp 990–991.)* Carbon monoxide is a common cause of accidental and suicidal poisoning. Its affinity for hemoglobin is 250 times greater than that of O_2. It therefore binds to hemoglobin and reduces the O_2-carrying capacity of blood. The symptoms of poisoning are due to tissue hypoxia; they progress from headache and fatigue to confusion, syncope, tachycardia, coma, convulsions, shock, respiratory depression, and cardiovascular collapse. Carboxyhemoglobin levels below 15% rarely produce symptoms; above 40%, symptoms become severe. Treatment includes establishment of an airway, supportive therapy, and administration of 100% O_2. Sulfur dioxide, ozone, and nitrogen dioxide are mucous membrane and respiratory irritants. Methane is a simple asphyxiant.

481. The answer is d. (*Hardman, pp 1549, 1641.*) Unlike Pb, Hg, and Bi poisoning, chronic Zn poisoning does not manifest itself by CNS involvement. It can cause anemia and thrombocytopenia. Pancreatic involvement causes a decrease in secretion of amylase. Fever is a common symptom.

482–483. The answers are 482-c, 483-b. (*Katzung, pp 1025–1029.*) There are many drugs that can produce significant adverse effects on the fetus when given to a pregnant woman. Among these are diethylstilbestrol, which has been shown to produce vaginal adenocarcinoma in female offspring. The incidence of clear-cell vaginal and cervical adenocarcinoma in women exposed to estrogens in utero has been estimated at 0.01% to 0.1%. Methimazole may cause hypothyroidism and congenital goiter by reducing thyroid hormone synthesis. Testosterone and derivatives can produce masculinization of the female fetus. Owing to low levels of glucuronyl transferase in the fetus, chloramphenicol increases the risk of "gray baby" syndrome. Sulfonylurea derivatives (e.g., chlorpropamide) can cause prolonged hypoglycemia in the neonate by stimulating excessive insulin secretion.

484–485. The answers are 484-k, 485-j. (*Hardman, pp 1061–1062, 1682–1683.*) Sulfonamides can cause acute hemolytic anemia. In some patients it may be related to a sensitization phenomenon, and in other patients the hemolysis is due to a glucose-6-phosphate dehydrogenase deficiency. Sulfamethoxazole alone or in combination with trimethoprim is used to treat UTIs. The sulfonamide sulfasalazine is employed in the treatment of ulcerative colitis. Dapsone, a drug that is used in the treatment of leprosy, and primaquine, an antimalarial agent, can produce hemolysis, particularly in patients with a glucose-6-phosphate dehydrogenase deficiency.

Ethylene glycol, an industrial solvent and an antifreeze compound, is involved in accidental and intentional poisonings. This compound is initially oxidized by alcohol dehydrogenase and then further biotransformed to oxalic acid and other products. Oxalate crystals are found in various tissues of the body and are excreted by the kidney. Deposition of oxalate crystals in the kidney causes renal toxicity. Ethylene glycol is also a CNS depressant. In cases of ethylene glycol poisoning, ethanol is administered to reduce the first step in the biotransformation of ethylene glycol and, thereby, prevent the formation of oxalate and other products.

486–487. The answers are 486-j, 487-a. (*Katzung, p 1029.*) Practically every drug has warnings concerning administration during pregnancy.

Most warn of the increased risk of deformities of limb development and defects like cleft palate. A few drugs carry the risk of distinct organ defects. For example, chlorambucil may cause agenesis of the fetal kidneys. Penicillamine seems to affect fetal connective tissue, causing relaxation of the skin, hypotonia, and hyperflexion of the hips and shoulders.

488–489. The answers are 488-d, 489-h. *(Katzung, pp 108–112, 1020.)* Atropine blocks muscarinic cholinergic transmission in the brain and in the autonomic nervous system. The result is dry mouth, thirst, dry and hot skin, tachycardia, urinary retention, ataxia, restlessness, excitement, and hallucinations, followed by stupor, delirium, respiratory depression, coma, and death.

Salicylate or aspirin overdose is characterized by tinnitus, confusion, rapid pulse rate, and increased respiration. The decreased partial pressure of arterial CO_2 (P_{CO_2}) plus increased fixed acids first cause alkalosis, which is followed by metabolic acidosis, dehydration, and loss of fixed bases. The picture may resemble diabetic acidosis, but the history of salicylate ingestion and blood salicylate levels above 540 mg/100 mL clinch the diagnosis.

490. The answer is b. *(Hardman, pp 1324, 1668. Katzung, p 1009.)* Deferoxamine is the treatment of choice in acute Fe overload when the plasma concentration of Fe exceeds the total Fe binding capacity. It has a high affinity for loosely bound Fe in Fe-carrying proteins such as ferritin, hemosiderin, and transferrin. The metal complex is excreted in the urine.

List of Abbreviations and Acronyms

α—alpha
A. lumbricoides—*Ascaris lumbricoides*
ABVD—adriamycin, bleomycin, vinblastine, and decarbazine
ACE inhibitor—angiotensin-converting enzyme inhibitor
acetyl-CoA—acetylcoenzyme A
ACh—acetylcholine
AChE—acetylcholinesterase
ACTH—adrenocorticotropic hormone
ADD—attention-deficit disorder
ADH—antidiuretic hormone [vasopressin (VP)]
ADHD—attention deficit hyperactivity disorder
ADP—adenosine 5′-diphosphate
AF—atrial fibrillation
AHD—arteriosclerotic heart disease
AIDS—acquired immunodeficiency syndrome
Al—aluminum
Al(OH)$_3$—aluminum hydroxide
ALG—antilymphocyte globulin
AMP—adenosine monophosphate
ANS—autonomic nervous system
APAP—acetaminophen (*N*-acetyl-para-aminophenol)
As—arsenic
aspirin—acetylsalicylic acid
ATP—adenosine triphosphate
ATPase—adenosine triphosphatase
Au—gold
AUC—area under the (blood concentration-time) curve
AV—atrioventricular
β—beta
B. fragilis—*Bacteroides fragilis*
BAL—British antilewisite (dimercaprol)
BCG vaccine—Bacille bilié de Calmette-Guérin vaccine
Bi—bismuth

273

BPH—benign prostatic hypertrophy
BPM—breaths per minute; beats per minute
BUN—blood urea nitrogen
C—mean plasma concentration
C_{max}—maximum plasma concentration
C_{min}—minimum plasma concentration
C. albicans—*Candida albicans*
C. botulinum—*Clostridium botulinum*
C. difficile—*Clostridium difficile*
C. jejuni—*Campylobacter jejuni*
C. neoformans—*Cryptococcus neoformans*
Ca—calcium
Ca^{2+}—calcium divalent cation
CaG—calcium gluconate
cAMP—adenosine 3′,5′-cyclic monophosphate (cyclic AMP)
$CaNa_2EDTA$—edetate calcium disodium
CCNS—cell-cycle-nonspecific
CCS—cell-cycle-specific
Cd—cadmium
CD—cluster of differentiation
cGMP—guanosine 3′5′-cyclic monophosphate (cyclic GMP)
CHF—congestive heart failure
CK—creatine kinase
Cl—chloride
Cl—chlorine
CL_{total}—total body clearance
cm—centimeter
Cn—cyanide
CNS—central nervous system
CO—carbon monoxide
CO_2—carbon dioxide
COMT—catechol-O-methyltransferase
COPD—chronic obstructive pulmonary disease
corticotropin—adrenocorticotropic hormone (ACTH)
CRF—corticotropin-releasing factor
CSF—cerebrospinal fluid
δ—delta
D_2—dopamine receptor

D. latum—*Diphyllobothrium latum*
DHT—dihydrotestosterone
DM—dopamine (3,4-dihydroxyphenylethylamine)
DMMS—drug-metabolizing microsomal system
DNA—deoxyribonucleic acid
dopa/DOPA/Dopa—(3,4-dihydroxyphenylalanine)
DTIC—dacarbazine
DVT—deep-vein (venous) thrombosis
E. coli—*Escherichia coli*
E. vermicularis—*Enterobius vermicularis*
ED—emergency department
EDRF—endothelial-derived relaxing factor
EDTA—ethylenediaminotetraacetic acid
EEG—electroencephalogram
EGF—epidermal growth factor
EKG—electrocardiogram
ER—endoplasmic reticulum
ETH—ethanol
5-FU—5-fluorouracil
5-HT—5-hydroxytryptamine (serotonin)
5-HT$_{1D}$ receptors—5-hydroxytryptamine receptors (a subclass of serotonergic receptors)
15-methyl-PGF$_{2\alpha}$—15-methyl-prostaglandin F$_{2\alpha}$ (carboprost)
F. hepatica—*Fasciola hepatica*
FDA—Food and Drug Administration
Fe—iron
FH$_2$—7,8-dihydrofolic acid
FH$_4$—5,6,7,8-tetrahydrofolic acid
FSH—follicle-stimulating hormone
FU—fluorouracil
γ—gamma
G. lamblia—*Giardia lamblia*
G protein—guanine nucleotide-binding protein
GABA—γ-aminobutyric acid
G-CSF—granulocyte colony–stimulating factor
GDP-GTP—guanine diphosphate and triphosphate
GERD—gastroesophageal reflux disease
GI—gastrointestinal

GM-CSF—granulocyte macrophage colony–stimulating factor
GMP—guanylic acid
GnRH—gonadotropin-releasing hormone
GTP—guanosine triphosphate
GU—genitourinary
h—hour(s)
H_2—histamine 2
H. influenzae—Haemophilus influenzae
H. pylori—Helicobacter pylori
Hb—hemoglobin
HbCO—carboxyhemoglobin
hCG—human chorionic gonadotropin
HCl—hydrochloride
HDL—high-density lipoprotein
Hg—mercury
HIV—human immunodeficiency virus
H^+,K^+,ATPase—hydrogen–potassium–adenosine triphosphatase
hMG—human menopausal gonadotropin
HMG—CoA-β-hydroxy-β-methylglutaryl-coenzyme A
HRT—hormone replacement therapy
IDDM—insulin-dependent diabetes mellitus
IgE, G—immunoglobulin E, G
IL-1, -2—interleukin-1, -2
IM—intramuscular(ly)
IND—investigational new drug (application)
INH—isoniazid
IP—interphalangeal/intraperitoneal(ly)
IP_3—inositol-1,4,5-trisphosphate
IRB—institutional review board
IV—intravenous(ly)
κ—kappa
K^+—potassium, univalent form
k_e—elimination rate constant
K. mobilis—Klebsiella mobilis
K. pneumoniae—Klebsiella pneumoniae
$KClO_4$—potassium perchlorate
kg—kilogram
KI—potassium iodide

L—liter
L/h—liters per hour
L. pneumophilia—*Legionella pneumophilia*
L-dopa—levodopa
L-thyroxine (T_4)—levothyroxine
L-type Ca^{2+} channels—L-type calcium channels (in muscles and neurons; have long, large, high thresholds of Ca current)
LDL—low-density lipoprotein
LHRH—luteinizing hormone–releasing hormone (hypothalamic)
LSD—lysergic acid diethylamide
LT—leukotriene
μ—mu
μg/mg—micrograms per milligram
μg/mL—micrograms per milliliter
MAO—monoamine oxidase
MAO-A, -B—MAO type A, type B
MAOI—monoamine oxidase inhibitor
MDI—metered-dose inhaler
mEq/L—milliequivalents per liter
mg—milligram
mg/min—milligrams per minute
Mg—magnesium
Mg^{2+}—magnesium divalent cation
MI—myocardial infarction
MIF—migration inhibitory factor
min—minute(s)
mL/min—milliliters per minute
mmHg—millimeters of mercury
mRNA—messenger ribonucleic acid
N—nitrogen
NM receptors—nicotinic-muscular receptors (found in skeletal muscle neuromuscular endplates)
NN receptors—nicotinic-neural receptors (found in parasympathetic ganglia)
N. americanus—*Necator americanus*
N. gonorrhoeae—*Neisseria gonorrhoeae*
NA—nicotinic acid (niacin)
Na^+—sodium, univalent form

NaCl—sodium chloride
NADH—nicotinamide adenine dinucleotide
NADPH—nicotinamide adenine dinucleotide phosphate
Na_2EDTA—edetate disodium
NaI—sodium iodide
$Na^+,K^+,ATPase$—sodium–potassium–adenosine triphosphatase
$Na^+,K^+,2Cl^-$—sodium-potassium-dichloride
NAPA—*N*-acetylprocainamide
NDA—new drug application
NE—norepinephrine
ng/mL—nanograms per milliliter
NIDDM—non-insulin-dependent diabetes mellitus
NMDA—*N*-methyl-D-aspartate (glutamate channel)
NMN—normetanephrine
NMS—neuroleptic malignant syndrome
NO—nitric oxide
N_2O—nitrous oxide
NO_2—nitrogen dioxide
NPH—isophane insulin
NPY—neuropeptide Y
NRC—National Research Council
NSAID—nonsteroidal anti-inflammatory drug (nonopioid analgesic)
O_2—oxygen
P—phosphorus
P. aeruginosa—*Pseudomonas aeruginosa*
P. carinii—*Pneumocystis carinii*
P. kellicotti—*Paragonimus kellicotti*
P. mirabilis—*Proteus mirabilis*
P. vivax—*Plasmodium vivax*
PABA—*p*-aminobenzoic acid
PAS—para-aminosalicylic acid
Pb—lead
PBP—penicillin-binding protein
P_{CO_2}—partial pressure (tension) of carbon dioxide, artery
PDGF—platelet-derived growth factor
PGE_1—prostaglandin E_1 (alprostadil)
PGE_2—prostaglandin E_2 (dinoprostone)
PGI_2—prostaglandin I_2 (prostacyclin)

PNS—peripheral nervous system
PO_2—partial pressure (tension) of oxygen, arterial
PPD—purified protein derivative of tuberculin
protein G—guanine nucleotide–binding protein
PTH—parathyroid hormone
PTU—propylthiouracil
PVC—premature ventricular contraction
RDA—recommended daily allowance
REM—rapid eye movement
RNA—ribonucleic acid
6-MP—mercaptopurine
s—second(s)
S—sulfur
S. aureus—*Staphylococcus aureus*
S. haematobium—*Schistosoma haematobium*
SA—sinoatrial
SAR—structure-activity relationship
SC—subcutaneous
SH—sulfhydryl
SL—sublingual
SO_2—sulfur dioxide
SRS-A—slow-reacting substance of anaphylaxis
SSRI—selective serotonin reuptake inhibitor
SVT—supraventricular tachycardia
2-PAM—pralidoxime
2-PAM Cl—pralidoxime chloride
T_3—triiodothyronine
T_4—thyroxine
T. saginata—*Taenia saginata*
tacrine—tetrahydroaminoacridine
TB—tuberculosis
thiazides—benzothiadiazides
TIA—transient ischemic attack
TNF—tumor necrosis factor
tPA—tissue plasminogen activator
TRH—thyroid/thyrotropin-releasing hormone
tRNA—transfer ribonucleic acid
USAN Council—United States Adopted Names Council

USMLE—United States Medical Licensing Examination
UTI—urinary tract infection
V_d—volume of distribution
VIP—vasoactive intestinal peptide
vitamin B_1—thiamine
vitamin B_2—riboflavin
vitamin B_6—pyridoxine
vitamin C—ascorbic acid
vitamin D—calcitriol {metabolite [active form-1,25-$(OH)_2D_3$]}
VLDL—very-low-density lipoprotein
VP—vasopressin [antidiuretic hormone (ADH)]
VT—ventricular tachycardia
W. bancrofti—*Wuchereria bancrofti*
Zn—zinc

Bibliography

Hardman JG, Limbird LE (eds): *Goodman & Gilman's the Pharmacological Basis of Therapeutics,* 9/e. New York, McGraw-Hill, 1996.

Katzung BG: *Basic and Clinical Pharmacology,* 8/e. New York, McGraw-Hill, 2001.

Index